F R E E

— **ONE** —

AUTUMN

DAY

ISBN 978-1-911079-18-7

Soundpractice

Soundpractice

Praise for One Autumn Day

What an inspirational read, I could not put it down. I would recommend that all healthcare professionals, be they nurse, doctor, surgeon, physio or medical student, should read this personal account of what it is truly like to be a patient.

Debbie James RGN
Advanced Nurse Practitioner

What an amazing story of courage. The phrase that stays with me is 'Battered, bruised, leaking but still here,' which can be understood by those that have been affected, either themselves or through their loved ones.

Dr Paul Fleet
FHEA FRSA

Fred Scott's book is an engaging, informative and candid account of cancer survival, and an invaluable resource for anyone affected by cancer. Through his personal story, Fred Scott reaches out to his readers and gives a rare insight on what it's like to face cancer and to navigate the bewildering medical environment into which sufferers are thrown. Highly recommended.

Dr Emily Salines

Many medical men and women gravitate towards their profession through some experience of undergoing treatment themselves or by contact with relatives in medicine. To some extent, this experience enables them to empathise with their patients to a greater or lesser degree. Nothing could prepare them for Fred's experience, as told so graphically here; nothing could provide the insight so movingly revealed in this roller-coaster ride through such an amazing life story with its musical accompaniment. We know so little about the dreams and aspirations of our patients as we pontificate about their illness, nor do we fully appreciate how our words can raise or shatter those dreams.

To some reading this book, it will not be immediately obvious that the author's survival is exceptional and largely due to the advances in chemotherapy, the effects of which are laid grimly bare in his account. Throughout the narrative, the character of the writer shines through and, to me, it is clear that his gratifying survival is, in no small part, due to his positive and dynamic outlook on life.

This book should be on the reading list of all doctors, nurses, physiotherapists, radiographers and, indeed, hospital porters. They will not only find it a most absorbing read but it will also enable them to "up their game" in the matter of their dealings with patients.

Mr A J Hall
Consultant Orthopaedic Surgeon, retired

One Autumn Day describes a patient journey through the initial diagnosis of bone cancer, through chemotherapy and surgical treatment, and the subsequent sequelae of such a diagnosis and ongoing medical treatment. This is an extremely informative and educational view from a patient who has had to deal, not only with the initial diagnosis of cancer and its treatment, but also the need to have further surgery to his limb. It describes the interplay between medical professionals, including the specialist nurses and the ward staff, together with the patient and the patient's family and their journey through the whole process.

The way that Mr Scott's love for music has been woven into the fabric of the book shows how someone's passion can help at the most adverse times. As a medical professional, I found this book enlightening and informative, and very moving at times, and feel it provides a great account of patients' experiences. I think this book would be of use for patients that have been diagnosed with cancer and their relatives, to be able to gain an understanding of not only the medical implications but also the emotional journey of a cancer diagnosis.

Mr Will Aston
Consultant Orthopaedic Surgeon,
Royal National Orthopaedic Hospital

I really enjoyed and was moved by your book. I thought that it was brave of you to relive all those difficult experiences and believe that it deserves to be truly popular. I did reflect that readers might find it reassuring to know that side effects are much reduced for most of the treatments given today.

Professor Richard Begent
Oncologist, UCL

It makes a great story, not only for someone who knows the whole system but I would think for an outsider. I think it tells the story well from the human side but also the technical things pretty accurately.

Dr Philip Savage
Oncologist, Charing Cross Hospital

I saw your writing as a sort of affirmation of life, but I didn't get the impression of an 'I beat cancer' book – but rather about how cancer altered and then became part of your life, and to this day, it's a process that has happened and now is integrated into your life.

Dr Nadine Izumi
Anaesthetist

Written in a compelling way to the point where one has to read it in one sitting. As a reader, you travel, along with the author, on his journey of traumatic experiences, peppered with humour and a practical, philosophical and spiritual insight into life.

June Perry
Editor, *Whitewater* Magazine

It is a very rare and privileged gift to be invited to glimpse someone's most personal struggles, loves and achievements.

Captain Jeremy Palmer

About The Author

Fred Scott is Director of Soundpractice Music
www.soundpractice.london

Fred is a composer, pianist and teacher.

He is married with three children and lives in London

Find out more about his journey through cancer here:
www.oneautumnday.co.uk

Dedication

To: Emma. My universe
L. E. Angel of Song
J. S. Angel of Strength
P. G. Angel of Grace

Author's Note

The fact that I am alive and able to write what follows is a testimony to the incredible work of the many medical professionals without whose expertise, care and attention over many years, I would certainly be dead.

My treatment in the UK has been under the auspices of the National Health Service. I am extremely grateful to this great organisation.

Charing Cross Hospital, Fulham

Mr Anthony J. Hall – Consultant Orthopaedic Surgeon
Mr Chris Schofield – Consultant Orthopaedic Surgeon
Professor Richard Begent – Oncology
Professor Edward Newlands – Oncology
Professor Kenneth Bagshawe – Oncology
Professor Michael Seckl - Oncology
Dr Philip Savage – Oncology

Royal Prince Alfred Hospital, Sydney, Australia

Professor Martin Tattersall – Professor of Cancer Medicine

Royal National Orthopaedic Hospital, Stanmore

Mr Stephen Cannon – Consultant Orthopaedic Surgeon
Mr Will Aston – Consultant Orthopaedic Surgeon
Dr Simon Warren - Microbiologist
Patricia McEntee – Fundraiser, Skeletal Cancer Action Trust
Nursing and ancillary staff of the Coleman Unit
RNOH Physiotherapy Team

Woodside Health Centre, South Norwood

District nursing team

Addiscombe Road Surgery, Shirley

Dr B. S. Jayaratne and his secretarial team

The Shirley Pharmacy

Dana Fathipour and the team

Additional Thanks

I would especially like to thank my editor, Leila Dewji, whose vision, gentle encouragement and inspiring commitment made this book possible.

Contents

Foreword
by Stephen Cannon

In his *One Autumn Day* Fred Scott, himself a talented and accomplished musician, portrays an epic journey packed full of peaks of elation and troughs of despair.

It tells the life-long story of a fit and articulate young man receiving a life-threatening diagnosis at a critical point in his life. What follows is a reflective description of his reaction to the news and the gradual understanding of its gravity. His portrayal of each new interface, be it with a general practitioner, nurse, surgeon or oncologist, gives a fascinating insight into the health service and its ability to care. It may perhaps inspire considerable periods of reflection.

In parts it is a gruelling read, as the effects of some of the most toxic drugs known to man take their toll on the healthy structure of his youthful body. During this terrible battle Fred finds solace in music. Specific pieces are selected for various components of the story, which produces a lightening touch to the overall tale.
In the end, it is a story of success, how one of the most vicious of cancers is conquered by medical and surgical skill and knowledge, and not least by personal determination. It is also a story of adjustment and change, which must even now continue.

Stephen Cannon
Vice President Royal College of Surgeons of England
Past President British Orthopaedic Association
Honorary Consultant Royal National Orthopaedic Hospital

Prologue: 1985

Music: *'Can You Feel the Groove Tonight?'* – *Con Funk Shun*

True story...

A young man, 23, gets told he's got a growth in his leg and it's probably going to be bad.

'Better not start reading any novels then…' is the phrase that goes through his mind.

Out of the hospital window, he sees the river where he used to row and the towpath he wouldn't run on again.

'So, what's going to happen then, mate?' he asks the man in the white coat.

'We may have to amputate the leg and you'll have to have some treatments that will make you feel very ill. Your kidneys could fail, you might go deaf, and we don't talk about getting better. We talk about survival rates. Oh, and your hair... all your hair is going to fall out.'

Then some cheerful chap takes a photo – in case the young man wants a rug (wig) made up later.

*****

2016

I thought it might be an idea to write about what's happened in those intervening 30 years; life, death, love, birth, faith, pain, indignity, tragedy, laughter – good and bad, guilt, total incomprehensibility and then clarity, varying degrees of nonsense, and not forgetting the best and worst of human beings with all their glorious foibles.

Some names have been changed for obvious reasons but apart from that, it's all true.

How do I know this?

Because it's me...

So here it goes...

Chapter One

Water on the Knee

Music: *Torna a Surriento – sung by Luciano Pavarotti*

It was an autumnal day, the air damp after rain and the foggy waft from the river Thames pervaded Bishop's Park. One lap of the park was the accustomed warm-up before starting out on the usual route; north up Fulham Palace Road, past Hammersmith Odeon, left over the bridge, along Castlenau, Barnes Common, Upper Richmond Road, left down Putney High Street, over the other bridge, then the home straight. In winter, shorts, no socks, running vest, the proper shoes, of course. In summer, four layers, topped off with a thick tracksuit, 11-hole DMs. My favourite run: hands bandaged, with the obligatory *Rocky*-style air punches. This was my time to think, as I carefully dodged the dog-walking Dames of Barnes, as large as their toy dogs were small.

Back at home, a scalding bath, followed by my own homemade recipe, lovingly prepared in advance, Bolognese, a baguette, bottle of cheap Valpolicella and Pavarotti's *Favourite Neapolitan Songs* blasting through the Walkman.

It was on one of these runs that I had noticed the start of a nagging pain in my left knee, irritating more than anything else. *'Punch through it, run it off!'* Running, swimming and the gym were my way of doing something other than piano practice. Having been at the Royal Academy of Music since 1979, and

1

admittedly the least likely person to have become a classical music student from my background (that comes later), things with music were getting serious – I'd made my London concerto debut in 1982 with Beethoven's *Emperor Concerto*, done various concerts in and around the UK and overseas, as far away as Canada, and my music was being played now too; South Bank, in fact. Things were happening, and not too bad for someone who started late, at 14.

I did not breathe a word about the music side of things at the gym. Spending most mornings in the company of assorted doormen, bodyguards (ex-army), hard-men and heavy-set individuals, whose limited communications enforced an unchallenged anonymity, seemed somewhat oxymoronic for someone who spent his other time playing classical music. So, any dialogue was restricted to: 'You finished on that, mate?' i.e. 'Please move along, I would like to utilise those weights now, by your leave', or 'Mate… spot me, will ya?' Translation: 'Would you kindly ensure that I don't come a cropper with this bar across my windpipe?' Very different from what I would be hearing later in the day up at Marylebone Road: 'Ah, yes, Mozart! The phrase must sing, you must sing with your fingers, SING!'

The intersection of these two worlds was the increasing pain in my left knee, and now especially whenever it happened to touch the underside of the piano. Between that and the running, I started noticing the beginnings of a warmer than usual, warmer than strictly comfortable, and certainly non-ignorable swelling. Hitherto able to sleep through any circumstance, I was regularly being woken up by intense throbbing in that left knee. The familiar mantras of: 'No pain, no gain', 'Pain is a state of mind', 'It's only pain', count mantras, not sheep. Still, this couldn't interfere with the regular runs and so on it went. More runs, more swims, more gym and through it, the nagging pain; more than nagging, rather, enveloping, rhythmic and seeming much worse by night. I started to spend more of the night-time in a big, empty space occupied only by pain and me, pain that encroached now into dreams, half-sleep.

An interesting observation I was beginning to make was that no matter how many runs and how much weight I tried to pile on for squats or leg-presses, I was actually seeing the muscles diminish now, but the swelling around that knee was growing, and pulsing as it grew, going up the scale from plum to orange to grapefruit. In the 80s, a man could get away with wearing tracksuits or loose-fitting trousers. I needed that so that this alien lump was known only to me.

I began to realise that I had to talk about this with some of the chaps, and ended up having the typical mono-syllabic exchange of grunts appropriate to male conversations about, well, anything;

'Y'all right?'

'Nah, knackered me knee.'

'Iced it?'

'What?'

'Frozen peas, mate. Ice it'

A miracle! The relief from a bag of frozen peas: one of nature's great pain-killers. But when the heat from the lump had overcome the freezing effect, I realised that I should perhaps expand the number of syllables in my conversations and find another opinion.

'Yes, classic over-training. And what is it you're training for exactly?'

Well, I was doing all this as an antidote to hours of solitary practice but my answer was:

'Because I need to be in peak condition, sharp in body and mind.'

'Soft tissue inflammation, water on the knee. Rest it, cut down on the training. That should sort it out.'

Two or three sporting types later, I went to our family GP. By this time, I was in constant pain, lump throbbing away all the time now and me getting grumpier with it. In truth, the thought of anything being seriously wrong never even entered my mind, but I wanted to see what this was. After a first meeting and a repeat of the 'soft tissue inflammation' idea, I was asking myself why something called 'soft' was in reality bone-hard, pulsating, growing and by now, the muscles of the left thigh were beginning to shrink away. I went back to the GP and insisted that I wasn't going to leave without an X-ray being requested by him.

That was how I ended up at Charing Cross Fracture Clinic.

The Cross, a large, unsurprisingly cruciform building dominates that part of Fulham Palace Road, just before the Hammersmith flyover, and was very familiar to me. Not only did I run past it regularly and walk past it to get to the Metropolitan line to Baker Street, but two of my family members had a long acquaintance with the inside of the building, as patients; my father and brother had been treated there for Crohn's disease – a spectacularly nasty affliction of the gastro-intestinal tract, which is very rare to find in multiple family members apparently, though not in our case. So instead of running or walking past, on this occasion I would be limping inside, and as it turned out, it wouldn't be the last time.

Never having had an X-ray, I had no idea of how these things were done. I reported to clinic reception where I was told to wait for the Registrar. Well, I hadn't been on a register since the fifth form, this was going back... Turns out a Registrar, like many seemingly arcane medical titles, is a step or so up from Houseman and junior doctor, but lesser than Consultant. A Registrar can still be 'Doctor so and so'. It's good to learn that the big cheeses are the 'Misters'; the Martial Arts Masters who, after having completed every level of bare-handed mayhem, wear a white belt once again.

So, the Registrar, Dr (now Mr) Schofield and I have our discussion about sport and water on the knee. He has a quick look at the lump, feels it, remarks with his eyes and a slight tilt of the head, which I read as surprise. Adrenaline can have that effect, especially in hospitals; every gesture takes on some or other connotation, intended or not. Doctors know this, I believe, and so are guarded, usually.

'OK, Mr Scott.' I'm thinking, Mr Scott is my dad, not me; they've already got the wrong bloke. I am Fred, always have been, sometimes, and only to my mum, Frederick, and if I'm in trouble.

'Let's get you off to X-ray. Please come back and we'll take a look at the picture, OK?' I begin to see that this implied interrogative doesn't actually seek assent, more likely finding out whether I can take and follow the instruction. There is no option here.

Thinking, X-ray, do these things hurt? I am instructed to undress, feeling a bit coy. Gym nakedness is one thing; it's competition time in that changing room, silent but everything is observed, compared. That was the way in the 80s and it helped you plan the next few workouts: 'Got to catch up with that other bloke's medial deltoid development in a hurry!' No one in this room is interested; I am a patient, an X-ray job. Lying on the bed, I am directed into position. A bit of yoga, things are looking up! A heavy black apron is placed (not all that gently) on my lower abdomen. As I am thinking what on earth this might be, I am told, 'And this is a gonad shield.' My startled look of incomprehension prompts further explanation: 'To protect your reproductive organs from the radiation.' I derive no actual comfort from this, surprisingly, simply the growing realisation that radiation is

5

about to be passed through me. At any level to the uninitiated, that's got to be a worry! The technician retreats behind a screen. 'And hold it, and breathe in... (Whirring, clicking, whirring descending in pitch)... and breathe away. Dress up please, are you going back to the clinic?' Ah, I'm thinking, an open-ended question, and what if I say 'Nah, I'm out of here', knowing that I cannot leave the Registrar alone with this X-ray. It turns out that, after waiting for a few minutes, I am the courier of that very film in its big brown envelope. Shall I have a peek at this in the gents? It's a picture of me, it's mine, part of me's on that, why not, I think, and not for the last time, I am NOT looking at this, that or any other thing like it. Far too much information. How's that going to help me? Maybe waste my time, but not help me. That's for the doc, his thing. Probably show to his student doctors, for a test.

So, after an animated inner dialogue, I duly limp the film back to Dr Schofield. He takes it away for a look, without me. I feign disinterestedness and stretch out on a chair, relaxed in body language if not in racing thought, and with the nagging suspicion that I want to see that picture, knee throbbing as if in accord.

Featureless hospital waiting rooms of the 80s didn't have much in the way of diversions; today, we have plasma TVs, in-date magazines, papers. Back then, it was whatever scruffy *Reader's Digest* had been donated in 1976, and was extremely well perused. I was left with my inner world. Strange to say that nothing was coming into my mind, just the contemplation of the blank, off-white walls, lino floor, random bits of furniture, no one else around. Couldn't put together a single thought, no music, not even what I was supposed to be playing at a RAM concert that month; some late Beethoven, actually, the *Op. 111 in C minor*, not even the first notes, the dramatic descending diminished 7th octaves. I put it down to the fact that there are three of those descents; I was confusing them, unusual, disconcerting. I tried

thinking of the last workout, what had been the last thing I did...
had a shower, dummy! Just a hint of a thought that something
was going on that I didn't know about with that Registrar fellow.
What's the delay? He's gone home, forgotten me. I'm wasting his
time. Shall I just bail out? I'm not short of things to do. Going
away this weekend and...

And then he's back. No ceremony, pulls up a chair in front of
mine – since when does that happen? Hands together, fingertips
together and a penetrating gaze. Not one to back away from eye
contact, I return his gaze. My father taught me that you look at
the bridge of the nose, so that you're not oscillating between their
eyes, just a straight ahead return, until they inevitably blink. Any
thought of gaining an advantage here was somewhat undermined
by his next sentence.

'You need to come in.'

'Er... Come again?'

'You need to be admitted... immediately.'

'That's a bit strong for water on the knee, mate!'

'There's a growth. We want to take a look.'

'You've had a look. And I've got plans, what do you mean,
come in immediately?'

The hint of this being an outrageous imposition on my
personal arrangements, combined with the unblinking stare,
seemed not to be registering with this Registrar.

'Now, you say immediately. You also say "growth". So, what's
the story? What are you saying here? I have plans. I'm supposed
to be somewhere else, soon. I'm away this weekend. How can I do
this immed... what's the stor... what's the film all about?'

'Mr Scott... er... Fred, if I may? I've showed your film to a
colleague and we feel you need further examination. You need to
be admitted for that.'

'So you said, but...'

'We need to get a closer look at the growth. It could be quite serious.'

Now, in all of this, and for a good while afterwards, I heard the words 'growth' and 'tumour' – no more mention of soft tissue or water on the knee, let alone training injury. Somehow, the stakes had increased. There was still one word that was not used yet, or for a while afterwards.

We discussed how this admission business worked; I'd come in with pyjamas (which I didn't use at the time, preferring the covering I'd entered this world with), a wash kit, and I should also advise my next-of-kin. The most disturbing part of that for me was the wonderful prospect of going home and telling my mother this exciting new development in my life.

There remained the issue of the weekend plans – I had planned to go away for a student house party and was determined still to go. The negotiation centred around the fact that I absolutely had to be back at the Cross by Sunday evening because I would be having surgery on Monday. Surgery!

'You said tests. You mean X-rays, don't you? What surgery?'

'We need a piece of the growth to analyse. It's called a biopsy.'

Ah, now the use of medical terminology. I hadn't heard this kind of language since O-level biology. Some of those words started coming back to me; cytoplasm, Golgi apparatus, mitochondria, islets of Langerhans, and now a new one to add, biopsy.

I had now acquired a six-figure hospital number, remembered to this day. It was to become to me all that I felt I was, after all that was 'Fred' had been almost extinguished.

Well, I limp-walked out of the Cross, turning left to go home. It was about a mile and I felt every step of it. I had time to feel anew that grinding throb in the left knee. The thought crossed my mind to run it back, generate a sweat. I didn't want to get home before I'd thought about how to tell my mother all this. She'd already been through years of health scares with my father and brother, some of these at the Cross, but they'd made it, and whatever this biopsy turned out to be was all about I intended to get out of there too, whatever that would mean. I clearly had no idea.

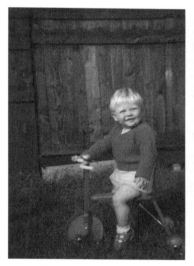

*Early years in Walthamstow
Ca. 1962*

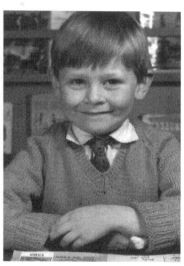

*Munster Road Primary School,
Fulham ca. 1965*

'I could do irreparable damage to a cup of tea right now. Anyway, that hospital thing – they want me to go in for a test... Yes, stay in... I don't know... I'm going away 'til Sunday night... yes, I want to... then I'm in... I don't know really... some biopsy.'

We were not a family that emoted over things, particularly not an innocuous knee swelling. Even to the extent that a hospital stay did not appear to approach the threshold of alarm. Those particular bells would chime later.

After all, my parents were of the World War Two generation; having met in the London Underground in the early 1940s, when stations doubled as bomb shelters, they married in a registry office in 1941. My mother's family were true cockneys from Shoreditch, working in the flower trade at Covent Garden. My father started out as a salesman for Munro's Flowers, later moving into the company's management. The old sepia photos from their wedding show the happy and smiling young couple surrounded by their parents. They went on to have a family of four, each child born after a gap of two years. The family was complete until 12 years later, when I came along as a total surprise. Typical of their generation of wartime survivors, they were never easily bothered by life events to any significant degree. My return from the hospital that day and my news barely made a blip on their radar.

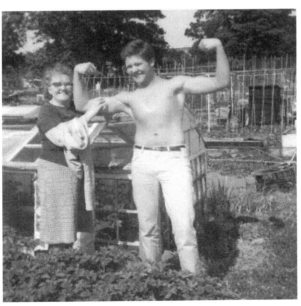

Happier days gardening with my mum in Fulham 1984

*****

What I can remember of the party weekend is restricted to the reactions of people to my news of hospital, X-ray, growth, and biopsy. Friends had a range of reactions. To some, this would be a chance to sleep and get free food, be nursed and not have to worry about washing clothes. This I could not understand, since I fully intended to walk out of that hospital as soon as they'd taken their bit of lump to look at. I was not planning on staying in any longer than strictly necessary.

Some students of a more medical persuasion seized on the words 'growth' and 'biopsy' with a little too much interest for my liking, and the conversations turned to the definitions and implications of the terms in a 'clinical context'. This was all very impressive to me, in a strictly pianistic context.

It was very easy for medical student friends of mine, with well-meaning enthusiasm, to give me a full rundown about what they thought this all pointed to. No doubt having heard about all this in lectures, it was time to flex those diagnostic insight muscles with me as the hapless 'subject'.

Growth became tumour and this somehow became **cancer** – interestingly not used at the Cross the day I was there.

Now, when that word, the 'C' word, the 'Big C' comes into the equation, it is a game-changer, and probably always will be. Cancer as a concept. Cancer as something that is to be dreaded. Cancer, the synonym for all that is fearful.

Cancer always happens to someone else. Somehow, I was now the *de facto* object of a new perception – it was obvious that it had been decided by circumstances that I was now associated personally with... cancer.

It is staggering how the perception of others can have an impact on you at this point. You are the one with the growth, whatever you want to call it. It is here that you begin to see played out in other people's faces and body language the entire panoply of human reactions. Bearing in mind there was no official diagnosis of anything more than a lump that was to be biopsied. The mere fact of a stay in hospital seemed enough for some to connect the dots and advise me that it had to be serious; it had to be more than a running injury. Maybe it was a cancerous growth (this suggestion coming from a non-medic with a streak of the morbid). This opened up a can of worms; was it something in your past, have you caught this somehow, is this punishment on you for being a cocky so-and-so?

My thought, in paraphrase: your concern is noted, your suggestions as to the cause will have to be ignored in the light of further evidence being needed before such a determination.

I didn't particularly enjoy this much. I felt that I was the object of hushed talk. Subjects obviously and rapidly changing when I was around.

Part of me wanted to confront this and deal with the suspicion and shift of attitudes. After all, I didn't have any concrete evidence that anything dire was in the offing and I couldn't afford to entertain the speculations of others. However, with a growing feeling of foreboding mixed with resolve, acknowledging a certain reserve in the 'Goodbyes', I left for London, back to the Cross.

Chapter Two

An Ending and a Beginning

Music: L. Van Beethoven; Piano Sonata in C minor, Op.111 – played by Wilhelm Kempff

Reporting to the surgical ward as agreed, it was late evening by now.

I walked into that place with no idea of what would be happening next or what would be different by the time I had come round after the biopsy.

An almost empty ward with one other man in it – a Greek family man – surrounded by his nearest and dearest.

Since a pianist of necessity spends the majority of their time alone, this was no hardship for me, particularly if people, friends, were going to act weirdly around me. In the quiet of that hospital on that Sunday evening, I had some time to go over recent events and take stock of where things were.

So here I was, completely alone, weighing it all up. I had a similar feeling to when I was about to go on stage and play a concert. In those moments before you appear at the piano, there is what seems like an extended period of cold analysis. Once you are seated in front of the instrument, there's nothing to do but get on with it. Fear is what happens before you're in a difficult situation. Courage only comes in proportion to the fear you've felt. As George Orwell said in his famous book about the year before 1985, the world in which I was living, 'Ignorance is Bliss', and this was very much not the information age.

No mobile phones, smart or otherwise, apple was a fruit, as were blackberries, PC was the prefatory address to an Officer of the Law, and a mac was clothing for rainy weather. Even if I had the desire, there was no option to research anything to do with this business other than ask a nurse, who couldn't explain much. Apparently, the Consultant would see me in the morning. I was instructed not to eat or drink anything at all from now on. A great comfort. So, might as well sleep. I lay on my right side and the old throb of the left knee kicked off when it touched the mattress, as if to remind me why I was here.

*****

To me, the process of being prepared for an operation was very efficient, no messing about. The anaesthetist came to tell me that he'd be putting me under, and bringing me back afterwards.

It was at this point that I met the main man – Consultant Orthopaedic Surgeon, Mr Anthony J. Hall. It is said that you can define a man by the company he keeps, or indeed by those who are following him. If that is the case, and by that definition, Mr Hall was a very singular individual. The epitome

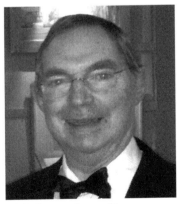

My first orthopaedic surgeon, Mr Anthony Hall to whom I owe my life

of authority in a blue pin-stripe, he explained to me in an affable but serious tone how this was going to work, while his team stood at a respectful distance, earnestly taking notes, alert to any comment he might make to them. I'd never had any personal contact with a surgeon of the order of Mr Hall, and his manner was a greatly reassuring influence. I felt that this part of things, at least, would be fine if he was involved in it. Apparently, the biopsy involved removing a sample of bone from the lump. I would then need to use crutches to get around, keeping weight off the leg as it would be unstable. In the meantime, the pathology lab would determine if the team's suspicions as to the nature of the lump were justified.

Never having had a general anaesthetic before, I had no idea how this all worked.

I remember waking up, seeing a vague daylight and being unable to move, trying to say something and hearing a strange, unfamiliar babble come out.

'Are you OK, Fred?' said a distant voice in a nurse's lilt.

Far from OK, as it turned out. A hitherto unaccustomed degree of pain was shooting up from my left knee and I could just about manage a slightly outraged 'Wh-hoa! What's with that pain?'

A wave of warmth took that away sharpish, then the lilt again. 'Just given you something for the pain, Fred,' and whatever that was, it was the business!

Eventually, during the course of what I supposed were a couple of hours, I became aware that I was up on a different surgical ward next to a window. Trying to sit up, accompanied by the complaints of what seemed a totally immobile leg, was an interesting new challenge but with help, I managed it – and then wished I hadn't.

Looking out of the window, I could see the Thames just south of Hammersmith Bridge, the very towpath that our school rowing teacher used to ride along as we dragged ourselves back to the boathouse from a row up to Chiswick.

*****

After passing the required entrance exam, my secondary education had been under the auspices of St Clement Danes Grammar School, DuCane Road. Situated near Wormwood Scrubs prison, the school had a reputation as a fine establishment in the 'old-style' – plenty of ex-military types teaching with the kind of rigour and discipline you'd expect. As an 11 year old, you felt it a privilege to be there. It was an environment where you were known only by your surname, which you didn't want to hear called out too often by these men. My best friend from primary school, Gary, and I went on to Danes together. We're still best friends and regularly reminisce with affectionate nostalgia about the place. I was aware that I was enjoying opportunities not afforded to my much older siblings, all of whom born during World War Two. Coming along 12 years after the last of them gave me the feeling of being somewhat disconnected from their pre-existent family unit; they had all shared the privations of the post-war years of austerity. My parents, being that much older, were probably expecting easier years now that their children were grown up. They were unprepared for the considerable challenges of being mature-age parents. Inevitably, the fact that I had things generally easier than the others created some resentment. Visits from my siblings were fairly rare at this time. We were not a family unit that pulled together in adversity. One conversation in particular with one of my brothers has stayed with me, in which I was asked why I seemed so cheerful. It went something like:

'So, how long before they cut this leg off. And what will you do if they have to chop the other one off too? Where's your God now?' Cruel if it had been meant as a joke, incomprehensible given the context. I had always had some kind of belief that what we see around us isn't necessarily all that there is to life and had, about a year prior to all this happened, begun to think much more seriously about spiritual matters and faith in a 'higher power'. Some of my friends thought I had become 'religious' or that I was searching in that direction. As I realised during the conversation with my brother, who professed no belief in anything beyond himself, 'religion' is often the cause of irreconcilable division between people, mistrust, prejudice, even war.

I was fortunate in having a few close friends and one in particular, Melanie, organised cards and messages of support. In the days before social media, she was a one-woman network of encouragement. Later, she would prove to be instrumental in bringing me together with someone of eternal significance to me.

*****

'Come on you boys, paddle... FIRM.' I wanted to be out there now. This was also one of the routes I used for running. With a piece of bone taken out, how long before I could do that again?

As it turned out, I would never run again, and haven't... to this day. It was the end of innocence, going from having no real cares in the world, and now beginning to face up to the ultimate living nightmare.

It seemed like some cruel joke, but who'd want this to happen to me. Was it actually down to me? What was this payback for exactly? I was 23 years old and in the space of about a week, my entire world was changed, for the worse.

Another level of loneliness kicked in. I didn't know anyone of my age or circumstances to whom this had happened.

Everything was tied up with fitness; time to think, time to go over the music I was writing or playing, make plans, dream of the future, just to plain enjoy the scenery, the sweat, the feel of my heart pulsing away, the bite of early morning, calm late nights, peace...

This train of thought was confirmed as reality when a doctor came to see me and explained that when I was able to stand, after a going over by the 'physio-terrorists', as they were cheerfully referred to, I'd need to be on crutches, not putting any weight on that left leg and being careful not to slip or jar the bone. 'We don't want any loose bits travelling round in your blood, no nasty cells on the move.'

I didn't quite get that bit at the time; it was enough that I had to think about these crutches. Well, good for the triceps, was the thought I started to console myself with.

'OK, so when do I get out then?' I was convinced I'd be better on the outside than stuck in here.

'We can't let you go until we have your results back, I'm afraid.'

'I live half a mile away, are you serious?'

'There are tests we have to do, quite a few tests actually. We need to find out exactly what's going on, and we need you in here, ready for the tests.'

I realised this was going nowhere; I just had to submit to the process, they were winning. I was beginning to piece this together now.

'So, what tests? You've got X-rays already. Need more of them?'

Turned out that they were thinking this was quite serious; lump became growth and had now become, possibly, a tumour; a bone tumour, no less.

How reassuring that we were narrowing things down. Wish I hadn't asked.

I decided that denial was a good option. I trusted my body, let them do what they think they need to do and things will be fine. I'm strong. I train six days a week. I have a good reason to get out of here as soon as I can, so bring it on.

Days dragged on. Routine becomes important, some order, some way of measuring time in a meaningful way. In hospital, the rhythms of the day have always revolved around 'obs' (observations); blood pressure, temperature and the inevitable question about bowel movements. Then the unexpectedly welcome hospital food; I was tipped off that double-ticking the options menu meant a double helping, especially welcome in the morning – double scrambled eggs for that all-important protein.

Tests it was then, for the next week or so, on a daily basis.

More X-rays. Why they wanted pictures of my lungs, I couldn't figure out, yet.

Kidney scan – this was interesting; I was flat on a trolley with a big, burly, smiling bloke in a white lab coat. 'I'm going to inject you with a dye and look at how it passes through your kidneys; we're going to take some pictures.'

The largest syringe I'd ever seen, full of a deeply suspicious and deeply red fluid, was poised above a tube going into my arm.

'We call it Congo Red, it shows up really well.'

I'm thinking, surely that's not all for me, as the plunger starts to slide.

'You might get a funny taste and feel a bit hot, sorry about...'

Yes! Both of those things! Burning just under my skin everywhere and a vile taste in the back of my nose confirmed what he'd said. I felt like I was on fire, so glad it was helpful for the pictures. I later learned the real reason for the Congo Red business.

Next stop, the Gamma camera. Very sci-fi. I am sat in front of a large circular machine of about three feet in diameter and a foot thick.

The cheerful operator calls out to me, 'If you look at the screen, you can see your skeleton', and low and behold, there I am, just bones. I wasn't smiling but my skull seemed to be. This was just weirdness. They were mapping my bones; again, I wouldn't know why until later. Just stay in denial and enjoy the ride.

The mother of all tests was the CAT scan. Bearing in mind that this particular machine is now in the Science Museum as an exhibit indicates that things have at least progressed in that area.

I am placed on a trolley and wheeled into a room, bare except for a large, white metal doughnut. I am wheeled into the hole of this doughnut, told to lie still and wait for instructions as I am left alone with a faint humming coming from the machine.

'OK, Mr Scott?'

'Fred, please, my dad is Mr Scott.' If I establish a rapport, will they take it easier?

'Fred, then. Please lie still. It's going to be very noisy but don't be afraid. The machine will pass over your body in stages. We'll be here for a while.'

They weren't joking. This thing had no visible moving parts but something inside it was shooting left to right around this doughnut and making a noise that has now become fashionable as an essential component in dubstep!

Unbelievable! Rather intimidating. At least the Gamma camera had been quiet.

This was hot, claustrophobic and seemed to go on forever, the occasional gap for what I presumed to be a re-loading or something similar, then more of the same.

BONE SCAN - 4.11.85

The scan shows a very conspicuous irregular region of increased uptake of radio activity at the lower end of the left femur involving both condyles but mainly the medial and with some extension outside the line of the normal bone. Elsewhere the skeleton is completely normal.

The appearances are quite typical of an oteogenic sarcoma.

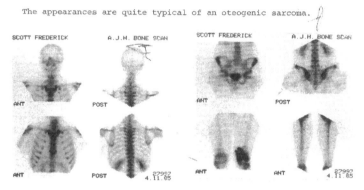

Gamma camera bone scan 1985

Eventually, it ended. I didn't know that lying on a trolley being tested could exhaust me like this. The mixture of these new experiences, general pain from the knee and a racing mind was wearing me out. Let me sleep, and deeply!

A generous glassful of Omnopon did the trick back on the ward. Interestingly, Omnopon, or Papaveretum as it was known, doesn't feature much these days due to its potential genotoxicity, or in other words, causing cell mutation. Good to know now, not at the time.

My notes from the time indicate that I was given this drug in combination with scopolamine, AKA the 'truth' drug. This particular cocktail was useful in another context as the drug of choice for certain interrogation techniques. It effectively renders you incapable of thinking straight, an authentic 'Happy, Happy' drug.

The reason for these tests was soon to be revealed by the doctors.

I wish I hadn't found out, to be honest, as it interfered with my policy of denial or 'what I don't know can't hurt me' attitude.

Congo Red – this was to determine the ability of my kidneys to eliminate toxins.

Gamma camera – to see if there were bone irregularities, other than in the knee.

CAT scan – to analyse your body's tissues for any anomalous areas or potential tumours.

'You see, Fred, we have to look for anything that might be related to what's happening in your knee. If it turns out that our suspicions are correct and you have a bone tumour, we need to see if it has already spread into other parts of your body, in particular the lungs. The kidneys have to be looked at to see if they can hold up under one of the probable treatments you may need.'

In essence, things were getting very serious indeed in my understanding.

*****

After 10 days, my parents and I were told that I had a malignant bone tumour.

The team would attempt to shrink the growth via chemical treatment and if that succeeded, remove the tumour entirely, and in fact most of the thighbone, or femur, with it.

It took a while to digest all that and I could see from my parents' faces that they'd had some extra words outside of my hearing. I realised that I had to keep my by now well-practised air of calm resolve, not react, and think of a good comeback. Notably absent still was the 'C' word. Cancer.

The word that was used, however, was sarcoma.

It even sounds malicious coming as it does from the Ancient Greek root 'Sarx', meaning flesh. Think of sarcasm (tearing the flesh) or sarcophagus (stone tomb for the devouring of the flesh). I am struggling to find a positive connotation.

So, I find out that I have osteogenic sarcoma, a malignant tumour originating in the bone, or in other words, bone cancer. There it was at last – the dreaded word. Sarcomas can be aggressive and can metastasise; in other words, change their state and migrate throughout your body, setting up their home elsewhere. In the lungs, for example, which then gradually harden and turn into bony tissue. The penny was dropping as to why I had all those tests now. We'd have to wait and see if it was on the move or not, and that's why they didn't want me to put any weight on this leg, in case I send nasties around from the operation site. Not that I was close to standing up yet, in any case, rather floored as I was by the recent news. My parents' reaction was difficult. My father had always been stoic throughout his own health challenges and I actually needed his detachment and resolved to imitate that; I thought it was a good family trait and very useful now. My mother, understandably, had a different set of reactions, recriminations and sorrows. Her own mother and beloved older sister had died of cancer, and here it was again, having a go at her youngest child. The bare grief was etched in her face.

I realised that this was one situation I could not rely on my parents to help me out of. At this point, you can begin to feel even more alone, the very people who brought you into this world being now powerless to make this go away.

The problem with having a serious condition is the knowledge that this has an impact beyond you. There is a deep-seated fear in people that surfaces when cancer appears on the scene; a feeling of utter helplessness. Wondering what to do for or to say to the person who's just found out they have it. If there's any advice I can offer to someone with a cancer diagnosis, it is this: that you may well feel alone as you've never conceived it before. What in the world do you say to someone who has cancer? This is why people close to you who have always had the answers now have little or nothing to say. The feelings of irrelevance are real for them. It may be they mean well but simply cannot articulate that.

Again, a visit from Mr Hall; this was something to focus on, the one person who could, in a blessedly dispassionate way, explain the plan without the steam of emotion involved. I needed this. A cancer patient shouldn't have to process the feelings of others at this point, wondering or worrying about how they might be feeling or coping. It's actually all right to be selfish, since you're the one who is being attacked from within your own body. All your resources of energy, emotional, physical and spiritual are required simply to get from minute to minute. Usually, in those days, cancer and death were synonyms. It was beyond comprehension to me that I could be a young bloke running around one week and then a cancer patient, a cancer victim, the next. Here's where the word 'prognosis' comes into the equation. What can you reasonably expect to happen now?

So, Mr Hall is back with the team. He has the same authority and this time, a little more gravity in his demeanour. It was explained to me that it seemed the growth was localised and that my best chance would be to remove the entire lump. The standard treatment for this type of tumour, in the place it was at the end of the femur, was straightforward amputation of the leg. However, before that was considered, and to ensure that the cancer would not spread throughout my body, I would need a course of chemotherapy over several months. If the tumour was seen to shrink, it would be likely that any potential secondary growths associated with that tumour would be killed off by the chemicals.

At that point, the tumour and as much of the diseased femur as necessary, maybe all of it, and certainly the entire knee joint, would be removed. It was explained that there was a possibility of replacing the bone and the knee with an artificial joint – a massive prosthetic implant made of titanium – if enough of the original thighbone could be spared in the operation. As I was hearing this, my thoughts had been racing as to when I might resume my normal life. In the course of this explanation, it all began to slip away. One thought persisted – I would be lucky to live in whatever state I ended up in. The next phase, after a successful operation, would be another course of chemo for several months to further obliterate any remaining cancer cells that might have been lurking undetected until now. Live! Would I even make it out of this hospital again?

My next visit was from someone associated with the oncology team. I learned that oncology was the branch of medicine that deals with cancer, tumours and the like. In a spectacularly brusque way, the mind-bendingly bad news that is the reality of chemotherapy side effects are listed. The textbook-style recitation is bewildering and, against my better urges, I am taken aback. In the overwhelming majority of personal interactions with medical professionals at this time, I had never experienced anything less than total sensitivity and understanding. I felt that I had to let it be known to the ward staff that I'd had a bad experience, if not for me then so at the very least a recurrence could be prevented.

My notes of 14th November 1985 show that this was in fact taken seriously: 'He was a bit upset by the abruptness of the oncology team. Otherwise, he seems to be coping well, and has a reasonable outlook. He now accepts the seriousness of the situation.'

Thankfully, the situation is very different these days. Resources are seriously devoted to counselling, advisory services, helplines and the like to make sure that anything you could possibly need help with is covered by somebody, somewhere. Indeed, entire advertising campaigns based around helping a patient through their cancer journey are more common than ever. This has to be a good thing. Back in 1985, you could say we lived in less enlightened times when it came to the idea of treating the person as well as their diseased cells. That particular conversation was not unlike being coshed with a blunt instrument. Very matter of fact, no empathy. Evidence, if I needed it, that I wasn't really expected to make it. Nothing to look forward to except horrible consequences.

The truth was, and is, that cancer is isolating; the solitary moments of despair and helplessness caused when you're disoriented by the diagnosis can tend to steal your ability to see beyond the next test result.

*****

Later, I meet Professor Richard Begent. Again, a figure of great authority and clearly commanding the respect of his team, he relates in a more professionally measured way the news about what chemotherapy is going to be like. Chemo was one of those words that had the instant ability to summon up a particular image. In my case, I had a spontaneous recollection of some or other documentary involving hairless individuals vomiting and looking generally wretched and hopeless. Maybe that wasn't the treatment I'd be on though. The consolation of that notion soon evaporated as the details emerged. I would be taken to the treatment room and hooked up to various intravenous drips to administer the drugs over the course of three or so days. I could barely understand what that meant. If chemo was an injection, why the three days business? It turned out that a patient is given a continual infusion of specific drugs continuously over a three-day treatment period. Hard to take in or fully understand. I was told about side effects. This was not a welcome list.

The drugs can make you feel sick; in fact, you'll probably be sick, quite a lot.

Eventually, your hair may fall out too, all over. You won't feel much like eating, won't be able to actually, and you'll lose weight. There may be some other factors here, like kidney failure, hearing loss, sterility, and you'll need to stay away from anyone with an infectious condition or even a cold (I'm thinking at this point that no one's going to want to be near me anyway, so that will be easy), since your immune system will be extremely supressed and you'll be open to anything. A cold could become pneumonia etc. This was grim.

Hearing the list was enough; the details and implications were something I couldn't even process. The discussion was not about what life might look like after all this but rather survival rates, how long I might be able to stand up under all this before my system simply packed up. The thought of a future that probably wouldn't come was obliterated by trying to get to the next morning.

The only thing that could possibly be worse than the descriptions of the treatments was the fear of what was coming – the first day in the chemo room.

One last visit that day – a cheerful chap with a camera. Did I mind if he took a picture of me? What kind of morbid… 'We do this in case you'd like a wig when your hair's fallen out.' That picture sums up how I felt at the time.

Numb, neutral, attempting a smile, not pulling it off.

Chapter Three

Death Row

Music: *Give Blood – Pete Townshend*

I was transferred from the surgical ward to floor six, the chemo wing, and was assigned a private room, which I came to hear was standard practice for a new patient's first night on the floor. I imagined this was to shield the newcomer from the worst parts of the wing; in other words, the sight and characteristic sound of patients who had been on treatment already. The rather melancholy view of the evening lights of West London prompted me to take a hobble onto the landing near the central column where the lifts operate. It was a very quiet evening and I noticed a young lady sitting near the entrance to the ward. I asked how she was doing and she explained she was a new patient on the ward also. There are not usually barriers to communicating with fellow patients – just an acceptance that you're not in this place for the tourism potential. We explained our diseases to each other. She showed me that her arms were covered in small red circles. Apparently, a mystery blood disease that was killing her. Chemo was the option of last resort. I wished her well and hoped that the treatment would work. I hope she made it. I had a growing sense that the world outside Charing Cross was the unreal place, not this enclave of mortality and pain. In that world, people walked around oblivious to the ubiquity of death and thoughts of finality.

29

It existed in films and on television and always happened to other unfortunates. Death as entertainment. To those experiencing an incomprehensibly personal proximity to the concept of their own end, everything seems trivial. Perceptions are sharpened. Most things that cause universal worry become nothing. If you have life, there is hope. If you lose hope, you die. It's a rather simple equation. There are many stages in a conflict with cancer. I felt that I was still on a losing streak but I was determined to show up for the next stage. These thoughts accompanied me to sleep back in my silent room. No good speculating about the next day. If I didn't get some sleep, it would be worse. In the dream state, I was back on the road, running.

*****

In the morning, I was in a wheelchair off to the chemo room in the oncology department. The wheelchair was one of the new perceived indignities of my new life as a post-operative cancer patient. If I had already a nagging sense of foreboding, this was only amplified by a trip along a bare corridor, which seemed to exist only to house a steaming great vat of liquid nitrogen. I remember the cold and a particular chemical smell that remains with me to this day, and is instantly summoned on seeing Charing Cross Hospital. I can taste that corridor still.

Met in the chemo room by a kindly senior nurse, be-wimpled and calming in manner, I was told that a colleague would look at my arms for good veins. The IVP (intra-venous pyelogram) urinary tract scan (with Congo Red dye) had shown that my kidney function was good for the elimination of toxins and so the first treatment could go ahead. I had reasonably good veins back then so there was no problem slipping a cannula (large needle) into my forearm. I was hooked up to a bag of saline that dripped away for a while. I didn't feel at all sick! If this was it, no problem, I could deal with this easily. I wondered what kind of horrible chemo drug bore the name 'saline' – there was a certain menace to it. I played with the word, 'Saline, saline.' No big deal.

I spoke to the main nurse. 'This I can deal with. It's not making me feel bad at all.'

'No, no, Fred. Saline is basically saltwater,' she was letting me down gently, 'just to make sure you're hydrated nicely for the real drugs later.'

I was not exactly comforted by this. I was clearly an idiot and she was showing me great sensitivity. Maybe my credulity would be a good attribute later on.

'So, what are these real drugs then?' I asked, trying to sound nonchalant.

'Well, according to your protocol, you'll be on an infusion of cisplatin and a dose of Adriamycin, both very potent.' Weird names, meaningless to me, but with a sinister ring to them.

The saline, my innocuous friend, is taken down to make way for a large plastic bagful of cisplatin, which after connection is covered in a black plastic bag.

'What, is it illegal or something?' I joke, weakly.

'No. It degrades in light, so we cover it for protection.' I'm thinking, oh great! Protect the drug, as it poisons me!

It takes all of about 15 minutes before I begin to feel that I can't swallow. This sensation turns into a feeling that all is not well in the gut department.

A bout of belching follows, accompanied by fairly copious salivation. Not long after this, and against my male instincts to the contrary, I call for help.

'Nurse, I think I'm going to be sick,' as pathetically as you'd imagine that sounded.

31

Hours of vomiting followed. After you've brought up the contents of your stomach, which doesn't take too long, somehow you keep going, dry-heaving. It's now painful, doubling-up painful.

An extra bag is hooked up via another cannula – metoclopramide, the anti-emetic, designed to counteract the heaving and sickness.

I'm taken back to a new ward. Looking around, I notice some empty beds in the subdued lighting. The other beds are occupied by men with similar bags hooked up to them. Every now and then, there's the sound of heaving and vomiting from another part of the ward.

It's difficult to comprehend but this goes on for three days. In the middle of this, a nurse appears with one of the largest hypodermics I've ever seen, full of a reddish-pink fluid – the Adriamycin, named after the fungus it comes from, found in the Adriatic, I was told. It feels hot going in. I attempt to throw up again, nothing left to come up. The metoclopramide starts to slow the retching enough that I can look around and even acknowledge the chap in the bed to my left.

'We call this Death Row, mate,' he said good-naturedly, and without irony.

We discussed our cancers. He had testicular cancer; or rather that's where it had started. It was now in his liver but responding to the drugs and he seemed cheerful enough, devoid of self-pity. The chap in the bed opposite was not hooked up. He looked like a skeleton. Yellow skin, hollow eyes, deeply sunk, mouth open, semi-conscious and breathing slowly, I was reminded of some kind of mummified remains. But this was a living human, however contradictory those words seemed in describing what I was seeing. Shock, and the inevitable thought of how long until

I look exactly like that made me look away – what I didn't see couldn't hurt me.

It was late evening, I noticed. After my new friend, Jeff, and I had drowsily agreed that sleep would be a good thing, I retreated into my inner space with the aid of my Walkman and Pete Townshend. This became the signature tune for this part of the experience. No associations about the giving of blood, I just needed the beat, the awe-inspiring drumming of Simon Philips, Paladino's supreme fretless bass, Gilmour's characteristic, busy guitar. Perfect accompaniment to Townshend's impassioned insistence. I dozed intermittently, coming round to heave again every so often. I became aware of a pressing need to go to the toilet. I was next to the ward's bathroom. This was to be a supreme logistical challenge. I had to try to manoeuvre my drip stand, black plastic-covered cisplatin attached and, without pressing on the cannula in my arm or putting any weight on my left leg, hobble on crutches to the toilet. I could, probably should, have called a nurse, but I had to be able to achieve this modest goal on my own to retain some sense that I had not quite returned to the infantile stage of life.

I managed to start off but reacted with incredulous terror to the unstoppable stream of bright pink fluid pouring from my body. Time to pull the red panic cord. The nurse helped me back to bed and explained that Adriamycin could do that and that my innards had not liquefied due to the actions of the chemo. A temporary relief. During all this, I kept re-visiting the idea, or maybe hoping, that it couldn't get any worse. But in reality, it continued to get worse.

Back on the bed, I felt that a hand had reached into my intestines and was squeezing hard. There had been nothing coming out of my mouth for a while, other than grey, metallic bile so now, whatever was left inside decided to exit another way. In my further indignity, I was reluctant to press the call button again. It seemed to be a final admission of helplessness now that I was proving to be incontinent. It is a moment like this that makes you wonder why nurses do what they do. I have been on the receiving end of unconditional care many times now and I cannot fathom the motivations of these outstanding, selfless beings. Suffice it to say, gratitude and verbal appreciation, though never sought, are a good place to start. I have no sympathy for those that give nurses a hard time. I include here the government, which pays them pathetically, nowhere even close to fair and proper compensation. In a society that rewards the undeserving so many times and even exonerates the venal and corrupt political operators we seem to hear more and more of, it is a travesty that the selfless servants who attend our needs in hospital are marginalised and scandalously underappreciated. This is upside-down. Perhaps an extended, anonymous stay in an NHS hospital might sharpen and focus the thinking of those who are closer to numbers and spreadsheets than human beings.

My fulsome gratitude seemed appropriate to me but entirely out of place. Nurses are professionals. I was babbling out of pure embarrassment; I shouldn't need help to clean myself up, like a baby again. This hadn't happened for 22 years. This was not me, the real me. I was strong, independent... I'd played at... I was a concert pianist... my music...

None of this mattered. I caught sight of the man in the bed opposite. Motionless, shallow breathing, not a flicker across the eyelids.

Exhausted, humiliated and slipping into dreams, I closed my eyes, hoping that music would obliterate what was on the other side of my eyelids.

✶✶✶✶✶

I woke up fully during the night and saw something I'll never forget – it was a normal-looking bed trolley but instead of a bed, it was supporting a coffin-shaped steel box. It was being wheeled by two silent porters past my bed, slowly. After it had passed and still looking ahead, I noticed that the bed opposite was empty. So that was how it ends, I thought. You're finished and they wheel you away in a steel box, by night, no ceremony. Death Row was an apt name indeed for this miserable place.

For the first time, I was confronted by the thought that I might in fact die. I had never contemplated death before, not death happening to me anyway. I had never met three of my grandparents who'd died before I was born, and had almost no meaningful relationship with my paternal grandmother, who had been resident in a mental institution until the end of her life. The whole business of dying was not something that I'd seriously thought about. It was only the sight of the steel box that prompted me to consider this. I had presumed that this treatment with drugs was going to sort everything out after a few days. If I had known how wrong that was, I might not have had the resources to carry on with it all. Something in me was urging me not to look ahead but just to get through the next hour, the next vomit bowl, the next toilet ordeal. As it turned out, the event that brought me out of this state was the hooking up of the next bag of cisplatin.

'Nurse, when do I start to feel better?' I asked, as the bag was being changed over.

'Probably not until a few days after your chemo finishes. How are you doing?'

'Oh, just wondering.' It wasn't long before new waves of nausea began to roll over me. Feeling hot and sweaty from deep within, heaving, producing only grey mucus again for hours, I was going beyond exhaustion and interestingly, beyond thought. This was not exactly unfamiliar territory; as a musician, you are used to entering a slightly altered state when you're performing, and it seems that you are an observer of what's happening almost as if it isn't you playing at all – this is the best! As soon as you become conscious, that's when you remember that you have an audience, hear the odd cough and lose the moment.

I used to feel that state also when running; your body is just moving, your mind takes off, you feel a great distance from physical reality. My lovely state of reverie was interrupted only by retching, and that's when the thoughts of death came back. I lost count of how many times I had used the bowl; almost too tired to reach for it, I had it perched on my chest. A load of noise and pain for such a tiny output of concentrated, foul bile.

I had some friends visit, brave souls! Entering a cancer ward when you're healthy must be an ordeal. The first thought has to be 'I hope I don't ever end up in here!' Understandable. I vividly remember their facial expressions. The human face is extremely good at conveying true, unguarded feelings. The brain unconsciously transmits its thoughts and reactions to all those muscles in a very direct way. I began to see what pity and dread looked like where before I'd only seen laughter and happiness. You don't need a mirror when you can read your fate in the faces of those who know you. Deep inside, I knew that I had to try my best to be light-hearted for the sake of my visitors. I had never experienced being felt sorry for in my life and it was deeply odd and uncomfortable. My default character was always confident, light, gregarious and loud. I had always felt in control, even recklessly so. This was totally novel and disconcerting, this being regarded as 'finished'. I could read it in faces and body language. When I was alone again, I retreated back to 'the space'. If I was going to die then it would have to be done with me fighting, not backing down, and certainly not reacting to what others were perceiving about my situation, hopeless or not.

I must admit that I briefly asked 'Why me?' and carried on a dialogue with myself. 'Why me? Well, why NOT me?' No one deserves cancer or whatever terrible affliction is being considered, but it can't necessarily be seen coming either. In the case of my cancer, osteosarcoma, it's rare. A GP will maybe see one in an entire career (last time I asked). I had no risk factors before the diagnosis, but all of the common factors that fellow osteosarcoma patients report; usually young, usually healthy, usually sporty, not usually diagnosed early until the 'lump' is unequivocally NOT a soft tissue issue or sport-related injury. How could I have stopped it happening? I couldn't.

Once having negotiated this ethical and philosophical thicket, I realised that a tumour was a part of me, just as much as eye colour, hair colour, skin colour, musical disposition, etc. Many things that define you are mainly genetic anyway. In particular, it is believed that osteosarcoma is down to a faulty gene.

With that realisation comes the understanding that this particular cancer is a part of you; it did not come from some malign outside agency. It was sitting in my genetic coding from day one and therefore was, to some extent, unavoidable, a question of when and not if. The why/why not me question is irrelevant. The real question becomes how long until this ticking time-bomb of a disease can be understood and researched until the point that it can be routinely tested for and eradicated before it causes so much aggravation. The only way forward is research, and funding for that invaluable research, with the knock-on benefits that the science would undoubtedly have. There's no shortage of cancer charities needing money, no shortage of people contracting cancers, and no shortage of the naked terror that the cancer-free have of getting it. You would imagine that this would mean no shortage of money pouring into medical research, treatment and palliative care… Well, unless there is a dramatic and unprecedented change in the levels of giving by the time you are reading this, the money is scarce. The disease however senses opportunity and is on the increase, relentlessly. My hope is that you are reading this as an interested but healthy individual, on the far outside of the whole cancer universe. But if not, I hope the following pages can offer some relief, maybe even some hope, and perhaps some solidarity in your own situation.

★★★★★

Meanwhile, I was coming to the final day on Death Row. After my three-day stay, I would be able to go home to recover before the next session of chemo and more of the same.

Now came an interesting turn of events – life on crutches, trying to negotiate my way around hospital corridors on newly-weakened arms. At least they'd taken out all the drips and various tubes, a feeling of slight consolation that I wasn't having to drag my chemo drug stand around like some evil twin. Feelings of being pathetic were prominent; it just seemed so contradictory to what I had previously believed about myself, and what I believed myself to be. From young, fit and strong, certain and sure, to absurdly weak, debilitated, exhausted, slow, shocked and quiet all in the space of two weeks. Any sense of relief that I was going to get out of this place overshadowed by knowing I had to come back and do it all again with more surgery still to come. I stopped that line of thought quickly; it was too overwhelming and too far ahead. I had to figure out how to get home first. How was I going to get on a bus, the legendary 220 along Fulham Palace

Road? I usually either ran down this road by night or walked it to get to Hammersmith Broadway for the Metropolitan line to Baker Street and the Academy. In the event, it was a mini-cab. Being driven. Unusual. I was not used to being 'taken' anywhere. A realisation that I was now dependent. Didn't like that.

'You all right, mate? What happened to you then? Football?' Innocent banter from the driver, and how I was wishing I could say a simple yes and carry on explaining the reckless but goal-saving tackle that led to it. Here was where I learned the awesome power of a word.

'Cancer,' I said, flatly but factually.

'What? **** me, you poor sod.'

I would have to get used to hearing similar sentiments. The key is not to personalise it but to accept that you represent an incomprehensibly dreadful state in which to be. I was on crutches, grey but still with hair, and so relatively normal looking to outward appearances. Crutches safely stowed, I clamber into the car and across the back seat; my left leg does not bend and it's a slow, awkward and humiliating process. Pulling away from Charing Cross, I am thinking about what I have left behind. A piece of my knee, pints of vomit, dignity, but also it starts to sink in that life will be very different. Potentially short. That was a big one for someone with no real sense of mortality. Would I ever feel good again? Would I walk when this knee heals up? What did they say about that? Do they really mean they'd cut my leg off? I didn't actually want anyone to hear or answer these questions. I decided it was best just to focus on the next minute. How ridiculously cold it was outside the hospital getting into the car. How hollowed out I felt. How hard it was to breathe. How cold my hands were, fingers unable to move. Not good news for a pianist. Maybe I wasn't actually a pianist anymore. Could I go to the gym again, would I see the inside of the Academy? How many people that I knew had any idea what was going on with me? I wanted to disappear and not have to deal with that. Just switch off and look at the shops. I knew them all, having memorised this route; after all, I'd travelled it to St Clement Danes School and back every day of my secondary education since 1972. It never once occurred to me I would ever have been making my way out Charing Cross Hospital on crutches, minus some bone and after major chemo. It had always been a place the 220 stopped outside on the way back from school. Now it was to become a permanent reminder and Pavlovian trigger for feelings of nausea whenever I was to see it.

*****

Coming home after the treatment involved a new set of adjustments. The short journey back from hospital assumed the proportions of an epic voyage, accompanied by cold and car sickness. Bleak mid-winter, as the song says. I hobbled indoors, everyone was quiet. I crashed onto the sofa, stunned, shattered and desperately tired. The highlight of the next couple of days was feeling like I could eat something. I had been advised to eat as much as possible to get ready for the next chemo sessions. My mum brought in what was to become one of the greatest meals I ever ate – a ham sandwich on white bread. I had never tasted anything so wonderful. It was a great mood enhancer and I could feel the gratitude of my beaten body for this humble offering.

Having had chemo whilst it was winter in the world beyond the ward, I was feeling the cold intensely, especially at home, since our house hadn't been upgraded with double-glazing. Strictly old-style sash windows, and draughty with it. Again, a major adjustment for me as I had particularly relished going for a run in cold weather – rain or snow a definite bonus! It was hard to accept that I might never do that again – just another to add to an increasing list of what would go out of my life, if I survived this part, which seemed doubtful.

Life seemed unreal as the few days passed before I was taken back to the sixth floor of Charing Cross for chemo session number two. I ate as much as I could to try and put back on some weight, realising that the next hospital stay would be a food-free experience.

No one familiar was on the ward this time, no one I recognised from last time anyway. There was same generic type of chemo patient – pale, transparent complexion, bald and puking. At least I still, for some reason, had hair! The thought that I had beaten the odds on this was double-edged. If the chemo couldn't kill my hair cells then maybe it wasn't killing the cancer cells either.

Almost anything can be blown up to epic significance on chemo; every muscular, joint pain or headache becomes a potential tumour, the cancer spreading out and going for the kill.

It's time to get hooked up for the next round. As if in anticipation, or out of some kind of instinct, my veins have retracted. The nurse spends what seems ages poking around in my arm, trying to find a route in for the saline drip.

'Your veins are on strike today, Fred!'

A bowl of hot water is brought in and I am told that immersing my arms in this will bring the veins up. I remembered that this was a good procedure to help warm up your hands before playing as well. Now instead of getting ready for performing, I was getting the veins receptive for more poison, then more sickness, more heaving, more vomit. Maybe because of my demeanour and previous experience, I was hooked up to some intravenous metoclopramide, the powerful anti-sickness drug I'd previously had. I woke up two days later.

41

Disorientated, I wanted to know what had happened. It was good to have slept through the worst of the side effects, but there was a surprise I hadn't accounted for; when I sat up, I noticed that there were clumps of hair on the pillow and strewn around the bed.

'Oh, yes, Fred. It usually takes a couple of treatments for the hair loss to kick in. Seems like yours has started to go. Do you think you might want a wig made?' Such an item, in my family's vernacular, would be known as a 'rug', and I instantly dismissed the prospect, as it seemed that another aspect of who I was would disappear, along with my knee, sports, dignity, future and everything else that chemo was supposed to take away. One of my favourite books was (and remains) Thomas Mann's epic music-based novel, *Doctor Faustus* – in a passage midway through the protagonist, German composer, Leverkuhn, is having a conversation with an apparition he takes to be the Devil in person. Explaining all the reasons against Leverkuhn's intended pact with him (genius in exchange for his soul after death), the Devil conjures up a picture of hell with a chilling image. He explains that once arrived, the new resident is taken aback by the scenes witnessed and exclaims, 'You cannot do that to a soul!' It is this sense of surprised outrage that I felt all the more as each new layer of experience unfolded. Perhaps a little like Dante's journey, if that's not too fanciful. I had performed Franz Liszt's tremendous *Dante Sonata* many, many times, and now it seemed I was living the descent into a bottomless hell of my own – the only consolation being that I was not actually dead and had not yet 'abandoned hope'. In some peculiar way, these experiences were serving to illustrate what was going on in the minds of writers and composers when they created works themed around this subject matter. A perverse comfort.

*****

Back home again, I was sleeping on a foldout zed-bed in my childhood bedroom. The ill-fitting windows allowing in a piercing draft during winter, a single electric radiator staving off the cold in our non-centrally-heated house. I had lost so much weight that I struggled into every item of clothing I could, including an old ski-hat. Cocooned like this, I retreated into sleep as often as possible. As to visits from friends, I had been advised to limit contact with people in general and, specifically, if they had any kind of cold, sniffles or the like, contact was forbidden. Chemo kills off your infection-fighting white cells and you're more vulnerable to anything that's going – more mid-winter bleakness. During one memorable visit, and as we sat and conversed weakly, I put my hand up through my hair. The look of horror on my mate's face was priceless as a great clump of hair came away between my fingers. I repeated this until I looked like the classic fictional representation of a nuclear disaster victim, and would have been great as an extra in the recent and terrifying BBC docu-drama *Threads*, about the aftermath of the Third World War. I was due at the hospital the next day for a blood test, and decided to stop off at the in-house hairdressers for a quick 'all-off' job.

'So, what can you do with this?' I joked with the barber. 'Er, not much honestly, mate' There was some embarrassment in this interaction, which I sought to diffuse quickly. Not everyone can instantly see the funny side of chemo. 'Yeah, I know, just joking. Let's have it all off, nice and smooth.'

Sporting my new 'Yul Brynner' style, I noticed for the first time that I had two large moles on the right side, which I refer to as my plug socket. And so now, I was an authentic member of the bald-head chemo club, all credentials in place. Thin, bald, sick, colourless, transparent, frail – the lot. On the ward, I felt that I was the real deal now. No need to try to hold on to what was gone.

*****

I was getting used to the rituals of chemo now – off to the treatment room, bowl of hot water for the veins, saline drip to hydrate me and then the black-bagged serum of death. The familiar onset of uncontrollable salivation, inability to swallow, sick bowl at the ready, and off for another round of vomiting. Curiously, no metoclopramide-induced sleep this time. Maybe I was resistant to it. Obviously, I hadn't been aware of much during the second chemo but this third time, I was fully conscious. I vividly remember one night after lights out, stirring in the small hours and imagining myself to be in a scene from the then recently made BBC TV series *Tinker, Tailor, Soldier, Spy*. One of the British agents, Jim Prideaux, is describing his treatment after capture at the hands of his interrogators. I fancied that I could relate and thought to myself, you will NOT break me! The 'you' was addressed to the cancer itself. I had no evidence to suggest that my treatment was going to pull me through, just a lot of puking and pain so far. I had gone beyond hoping for anything after all this. I was not even halfway through the process. Surgery was yet to come, and the joy of another three planned chemo sessions. If the operation was successful…

*****

Home again, with instructions to eat as much as possible, stay away from anyone with a cold. Sleep a lot. I was well used to the discipline of physical training and practicing so I took this seriously and realised that I had to be in good mental shape, if nothing else. At the very least, I could control how I felt about this. If I had started to mourn what was lost, I could feel that this would reduce my chances of making it – make the future, such as it would be, an infinitely disagreeable place to survive the journey into. I was only 24. Not much of a life story if it ended this soon, but at least I was determined to go out with my sense of irony intact. Take all the pride and dignity you want but leave the spirit, I addressed to no one in particular. To that end, I decided that I didn't want to know anything about prognosis, outcomes, statistics or anything related to opinions about surviving. I'd already seen in the faces of my family and friends the impact of knowing too much and assuming that what you were told was the way it would be. I adopted a course of ignorance; what I didn't know couldn't hurt me. It might work, it had to work – it was all I had to go with. I figured out that if a baby can come into this world completely helpless, with nothing, and yet live and grow then even though this was the end of at least a part of my life, perhaps, if I lived through it, things might begin again. As Roger Daltrey once sang, 'We've got to have faith in something big outside ourselves.'

Chapter Four

'We Can Re-build Him'

Music: *Training montage from Rocky IV by Vince di Cola*

I was back in Charing Cross, this time admitted to the surgical ward and getting ready for my knee replacement operation. To this very day, on my annual visits for follow-ups and tests, the very sight of the building as I approach along Fulham Palace Road is enough to induce nausea, hot sweats and a feeling of dread, even, it has to be said, in sunshine. Despite the fact that it's been refurbished, equipped with the usual ubiquitous coffee shops and their comfy chairs, and the fact that the clinical staff look too young for the job, I am tied to that structure by the strongest of bonds.

It had been put to me that this was a relatively new and somewhat experimental procedure. I had nothing to lose, I thought, since the alternative was straightforward amputation, so let's go with this op. I had many X-rays and films taken for the measurements. The knee itself (or massive distal femoral prosthesis, to be strictly accurate) was to be manufactured up at the bio-mechanical labs of the Royal National Orthopaedic Hospital, Stanmore. A custom-made, bespoke titanium unit just for me. I was following in the footsteps of Steve Austin, TV's *Bionic Man*. That programme was a must-see for my generation and on a weekly basis, the opening titles of the show announced with great gravity 'we can re-build him', after Austin had literally been smashed to pieces in an aviation accident. This interface of mechanics and the human body was now happening to me, albeit without the full-body procedure that Austin had endured. But that was fiction and what they were about to do to me was real.

Mr Hall, orthopaedic surgeon, and his team made a ward round, during which I was told about the procedure. It seemed that the tumour had responded sufficiently to the chemo and could now be taken out, along with the complete knee joint and as much of the femur as necessary. The prosthesis would then be cemented into place, long spikes being inserted into the bones for stability; all in all, a very lengthy piece of metalwork. I had no interest in hearing any detail beyond that.

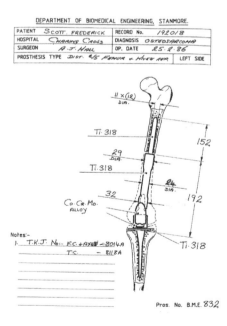

The Stanmore Prosthesis - original hand-drawn design 1985

Suffice it to say that I had never even heard of such a thing being possible, but anything was preferable to amputation, even though that was still an option if Mr Hall found anything nasty inside the operation site, or if something went awry during the surgery. I signed a consent form to that effect after this had all been explained. I completely trusted Mr Hall and on that basis, I mentally committed to the operation and whatever consequences would follow from it.

For the first time, I heard about 'Stanmore' – a mysterious place in North West London where the prosthesis was going to be manufactured. I heard that it would be delivered to Charing Cross by Securicor in time for the operation.

This all seemed a bit unlikely to me and I asked myself how on earth this was all going to work in reality. I had decided not to doubt what Mr Hall said and taking his word for it, I put my thoughts aside.

I took a pre-op mental audit; in an incredibly short space of time, my life had completely changed. Anything that I thought I was or had achieved in life was irrelevant. All the striving in music, all the ambition for a future in that profession snuffed out. My highly-prized fitness now gone along with it. An invader from within my own body, my own genetic code, had taken control of my life. It seemed like a kind of coup. It may be a cliché but I was in a battle now. This metaphor is definitely overused because it has been devalued in many contexts. I will however assert the right of every cancer patient to declare that they are indeed fighting for their life and that every possible means of support be given them in order to make it on their own terms. One may want to be joined in this experience by others, or desire solitude. Some will want to embrace fully all available sources of information about treatments and cures; others enter a state of absolute denial. I think the one common thread is that each cancer and each person with cancer is completely unique, and allowing them simply to be themselves in the experience is essential.

It was 25th February 1986 on ward 7 North and preparation time for the surgery. Not the first because I'd had a biopsy done before this but in my mind, that didn't count for much – this was the Big One. I had to sign a form to consent to what was termed 'mutilating surgery', with the possibility of amputation and the usual risks of infection, reactions to drugs and the like. I'd signed a few forms and the odd cheque but this would be the most significant signature of my life to date. The permission to knock me out with anaesthetic for about five hours, remove half my left femur, knee and the top of the tibia, and inserting the metalwork. I didn't want to see any diagrams, notes, pictures or anything else. I couldn't even conceptualise what it would look like afterwards. In truth, what was bothering me more was the removal of what the bone and associated components represented – my youth, my health, possibility, ability, mobility. This business of handing myself over was going against all my instincts and experience. As a pianist, I had become used to being in control of circumstances. You don't reach that level of achievement by accident or due to anyone else directly. It's all about how much time and effort you put in, how much control you gain, through long and laborious hours practicing, of your mind, body and emotion. When you go out onto a stage to perform, you are utterly alone, except for the piano, which you hope is going to be your friend and collaborator. You have to subdue yourself but coax the instrument. In the end, however, you are responsible for the sound and with it, the possibility that your audience is going to 'get' the music. You play the final notes, the spell is broken, by you, and it's over. You have been in charge the entire time.

The nurse brought me a small package containing two items of clothing, unparalleled in sartorial elegance. The surgical underpants, rather like the same material used for a string vest, and a surgical gown. My first attempt to put it on provoked some mirth.

'Er... Nurse. Not sure this is the right size. It won't do up and it feels really tight across the shoulders.' Now, this was not due to unprecedented development of the deltoid group but solely down to the fact that I'd tried to put the thing on back to front. Therefore, to my relief, amid embarrassment, I reversed the gown. It's supposed to cover your front and leave your back exposed. Much more comfortable this way. Then comes the long wait, curtains drawn around the bed. I was confronted by the total unreality of all this, and looking down and along my left leg, I felt a nostalgic kind of compassion for my beleaguered limb and what was soon going to happen to it. It might not even be there when I woke up.

You've done me no wrong. Why is this happening to you? I quickly dismissed that thought. I told myself that my only option was to trust Mr Hall. And I did.

After a while, a nurse appeared with a syringe on a tray. Having been 'nil-by-mouth' since the previous evening, I could have drunk a gallon of the neighbouring Thames itself, but the contents of this syringe were the only fluids I would see for the next several hours.

'Hello, Fred. I expect you're feeling a bit nervous.'

A couple of typically facetious comebacks flitted across my mind before I settled on, 'Yes. Not used to this.' Not strictly true as a musician is always nervous before performing, but that's a 'good' type of adrenalin buzz.

'Well then, this will help. It's what we call pre-med. You'll feel a bit woozy.'

There followed a quick jab in the fleshy part of the gluteus max, the intra-muscular route.

Let's just say that this pre-med was fabulous stuff. I would have agreed to anything after that, which is probably why the consent form was done well before. Essentially, pre-med is some kind of strong tranquillizer (in this case Omnopon and scopolamine) that turns off anxiety, which it did – completely.

The curtains opened, ending my drug-induced reveries (I had never heard music sound so great!), and Chris, the trolley-man, appeared. A jovial, proper 'cockney sparra' (strictly speaking, I don't think that Chris was born in the East-End, but sounded like it to me – more about my familial East-End-ness later).

'Awright, mate? Let's get you off then.'

I remember grabbing Chris's forearm and babbling, 'I love you, you're my best friend...' in the manner of the archetypal, comical drunk. I imagine that anyone who has to deal with pre-operative patients must be privy to the most extraordinary conversations. The proximity of oblivion can induce a profoundly confessional state in people.

On reaching the operating theatre suite, the trolley comes to a halt. I am by this time as high as a kite or freewheeling peregrine falcon, flying far above the slings and arrows, as Shakespeare put it, but not quite ready to shuffle off the old mortal coil just yet.

'OK, Fred. Sharp scratch coming. Just count down from ten, nine, eight, sev...'

Anaesthesia is about as close to actual death as you can probably get, this side of the real thing. A deep and dreamless state of helplessness. You are completely dependent on the skill of the anaesthetist to monitor your signs during surgery, making sure you don't wake up in the middle of it all, and bring you back afterwards.

The lilting sound of the recovery nurse is the first sound I registered on coming round. It's a bit like swimming upwards through a thick liquid. Trying to move and realising I was hooked up to tubes and monitors, I remember bit by bit where I now was. Still drugged up to the eyeballs, I couldn't care less about anything. Again, 'Fr-ed' – my name in two syllables and pitched in a descending major third (the same as a cuckoo's call). I want to answer but my mouth is stuffed with cotton wool and fur, seemingly. I manage an inarticulate kind of proto-speech. 'You're out of theatre now, in recovery, just rest, you're fine.'

I pieced together as much I could, thinking I'd come round after a particularly deep slumber. Yes! I'd had the operation on the... leg! I couldn't feel anything coming from the left side. I prepared myself in my mind for the fact they'd had to take off the whole thing. Sooner or later, I'd have to open my eyes, look down and see the damage, see what I was left with.

Shocked, I saw a huge white cast, covered in bandage, and surgical tape with tubes coming out from the top near my groin and about halfway down. These tubes were obviously carrying blood, in or out of me, I couldn't tell.

Eyes shut and back to sleep, taking in the fact that I had just seen the toes of my left foot, all still there.

'Fr-ed.' The call back again. 'How are you feeling?' It was more like singing, angelic singing, than mere speech.

'Mmnnaa,' I managed to groan. 'Mghaaa.' Roughly translated as 'I'm beginning to suspect that a world of pain is coming my way', and indeed it was. Not too bad though because it meant that my limb was letting me know it was still in place, however battered it may be. One of the side effects of being under anaesthetic for several hours is that you throw up. In my case, despite a raging thirst, I was somehow generating enough fluids from somewhere to vomit copiously. I was told that I'd be free to drink a few sips after I'd stopped with the puking. In the meantime, a nurse kindly dabbed my lips with wet cotton wool and even occasionally passed an ice-cube across my mouth. I wanted to swallow that cube but no amount of pathetic pleading prevailed. Hard-line, tough-love nursing. It was apparent that if I drank more, I would vomit longer. My mind was gradually becoming clearer and less obsessed with hallucinations of flying cups of tea, thick, brown, industrially strong and brewed to perfection.

The most common thing in the world, a glass of water, a cup of tea, a slice of bread, can take on an almost mystical aura of significance because they are denied to you in the immediate post-operative state. The gratitude towards that person who finally gives you the all-clear to drink is overwhelming.

Another sensation appeared on my horizon; I was becoming aware of a need to go to the toilet. I couldn't understand. If I was this absurdly thirsty and yet throwing up, how could there be anything in my bladder? Surely all available liquid would have deployed elsewhere? I tried to figure out how I would possibly get up and take care of this bit of business. I took stock of my position. Tubes in the arms, left leg heavily plastered, more tubes coming out of that, I was immobile too. Curtains were drawn around the bed so I had no idea of whether I was back in the solitary room. Some random noises and snippets of conversation let me know the presence of others. This didn't sound like the chemo ward. Must be the surgical ward. I was feeling more pressure and desire to go to the loo. And there seemed less I could actually do about it. I found the call button.

'Are you all right, Fred? You still can't drink yet, you know.'

'No, no. I'm just thinking what happens when I need to go...'

'Oh, do you think you might need a bottle?'

'But you said I can't drink...'

'No, I mean a pee-bottle. I'll get you one.'

Salvation! I didn't know these things existed. The bottle disappeared under the sheets, manoeuvred into position and relax, and...

Nothing. The longer I concentrated, the more tension I felt and the more the pressure grew in the bladder area. When the nurse returned for the second time to ask how I was doing, I had to confess that there was no output. Discussing with a young lady my inability to urinate was a new indignity. Surely there were some limits to these humiliations?

'Well, Fred, if you are really not able to go, we may have to use a catheter.'

I nodded with no comprehension of what 'catheter' meant. Maybe a different kind of bottle?

'We'll have to pass a tube straight into your bladder and drain the urine.'

'What, through my stomach or something?'

I wished I hadn't gotten into this exchange on discovering the intended actual pathway of the said tube. Typically male, I was squeamish about the mere idea of this proposed tubish intrusion. Never! I had to buy some time.

'No, I think it'll be all right. Just a bit more time. I'll stick with the bottle.'

I was strangely encouraged by this. Focussing on this logistical nightmare took my mind off the pain from the leg. I had to go to the toilet or face catheterization.

Discomfort soon overstepped the mark into real pain. Did I really need to add an internally-exploding bladder to my current list of afflictions? Then, probably spurred on by necessity, I had an Isaac Newton moment; it was all down to gravity. Those physics lessons from Messrs Crimes and Cardwell at St Clement Danes were finally proving their worth.

With confidence and resolve, I buzzed the nurse.

'Used the bottle yet, Fred?'

'Not quite, but I've figured out what to do. Can you help me?'

It is astonishing how feeble you feel after surgery. Weak and uncoordinated. My plan was to shuffle over to the edge of the bed so that my right leg reached over the side. Next, I asked the nurse to crank the bed up to its full height, my leg in contact with the floor and almost vertically straight. There was just enough play in all the tubing and cables to allow me to come close to standing. A little more of a shuffle, bottle in position. The moment of truth. Although not an authorized protocol for bladder evacuation, the plan began to work, all too slowly. The nurse understood this particularly male dilemma and allowed me the necessary privacy. Everything stopped again. This was becoming a mountainous challenge. It had to work or else.

I closed my eyes and tried not to feel the pain. Instead, I began to breathe rhythmically and deeply.

'Are you OK in there, Fred?' Back to square one!

'Nearly, just a minute.'

Back to the ritual exhalations.

On about the fifth of these, a blessed torrent resolved the problem to the point where I could barely hold the bottle. Tremulously, I called for the nurse. Exalted, exhausted, ecstatic. The relief was in proportion to the mountain.

This and many other small victories was a great morale booster. It is truly astonishing, the impact of something as insignificant as using the bottle.

It was up there with winning prizes, concerts that went well, all the rest.

I had conceived and executed an ambitious operation of my own. Some small measure of independence in all my helplessness.

Having celebrated my achievement with a little well-earned self-congratulation, I was less distracted by my own predicament and had a look around the ward.

This was a very different place from 'Death Row'. There were six beds. I was nearest the window and, once again, as if to reinforce what I already knew, I was overlooking the Thames. I had to dismiss the thoughts of regret. I couldn't even remember when the last time was I'd used that towpath. Questions were inevitably surfacing in my mind about the wisdom of setting any goals about getting out there just yet. I spotted a lone runner. Then, someone in a single seat boat, sculling along the river, away from Hammersmith Bridge. I had to ignore this. My reality was here and now on ward 7 North.

Opposite me was Mick. We greeted each other in the usual way common to males: 'All right, mate? What you in for then?' Mick was a despatch biker who'd collided with another vehicle and needed some surgery. He explained how, due to a chronic shortage of time on the job, he could stop at a traffic light, leap off his bike, shoot into the nearby McDonalds and neck a Big Mac down before the lights turned green. Even if this were a statement laced with hyperbole, I knew the location of this lunchtime adventure; Balham High Road, and despatch riders were the buccaneers of the road at the time, so it seemed entirely likely. In conversation with Mick, he explained how he was supplementing his pain medications with a certain smokeable, recreational substance smuggled in ready-made by a friend. I declined his offer to share in this self-medication, made in great generosity of spirit. It was little surprise then that our later evening conversation centred on food. Once I had recovered from the effects of the anaesthetic, my appetite was prodigious. My body crying out for nutrition, in the back of my mind, I was realising that I had to eat as much as possible before the next chemo sessions began. Whenever that was to be, it would be too soon.

Our plan was to call out to Perfect Pizza in Fulham Palace Road for an after-midnight food-fest. Fortunately, the nurses had no objections to this, maybe because we'd promised to share the goods, or more probably because they were superior human beings in the first place. About half an hour later, a tall, leather-clad and helmeted biker emerged onto our ward with the tell-tale large, flat box. The sight of that 15-inch pepperoni was glorious to behold, preceded as it was by the warm and comforting waft of hot dough. In my training days, I never would have eaten this but now, no such restraint appeared on my mental horizon.

Pepperoni pizza, truly the food of the Eternals; whoever invented that deserves the thankful recognition of the ages.

*****

The next day, I made the acquaintance of the man in the bed next to Mick's.

Like me, Dan-I had a leg in plaster and went on to explain that he'd been biking along Fulham Palace Road and a lorry ran him over, and then, as the wheel was on his leg, almost ripped the limb off as it turned to move away. Dan-I had received a monumental skin-graft, which he said had left his thigh looking like a crocodile, as he put it. Our friendship was truly forged through a mutual experience of pain. We were both on the list for physiotherapy. It is important to become as mobile as possible, if possible, as soon as possible, after an operation, especially on a large structure like a leg.

Even for someone used to a bit of gym work, this kind of post-operative physio was heavy-going. The first goal is to stand up.

The terrifying prospect of everything falling apart was very real. I felt phenomenally weak. Nothing worked as it should have. I could barely support myself on the crutches, shaking as I was. The physio team helped me to achieve another modest, but in some ways, monumental milestone – to stand up and take a couple of steps near the bed. Exhausting but exhilarating. My daily routine could now incorporate more and more adventurous excursions. To the end of the ward, outside to the nurses station, along the corridor. Eventually, around the entire floor itself. I was beginning to feel more like myself again in spirit, enjoying the camaraderie of my ward mates, late-night conviviality around a pizza, and the Five Nations Rugby on the BBC via the ward's one TV set, high up on the end wall, just about visible to all of us.

All the post-op signs were favourable and it seemed that I could be discharged home until re-admission for the next chemo session.

✳✳✳✳✳

Being at home meant existing between two rooms – my bedroom and the living room – where I had come to use the old sofa as a kind of day bed. Getting up and down the stairs between these rooms was not something I wanted to do too often. One trip up and down was exhausting, and somewhat dangerous as I had to negotiate the stairs on crutches without putting any weight on the left leg. Watching TV during the day became irritating. People have always asked throughout the ages if there is 'more to life than this'. I was aware of entertainment as anaesthetic that could help you to pass time. I suppose I was longing to go back to the banality of life before cancer. I had truly forgotten how I used to think about life, the concerns I had before seemed all too trivial.

My pre-discharge instructions were to keep the new joint as mobile as possible and show up for outpatient hydrotherapy. I'd developed a radical antipathy to the word therapy by now, but this hydro stuff was fine; basically you are in a conveniently over-heated swimming pool and led through exercises that provide some resistance to strengthen the insulted muscles of the thigh. I liked these aquatic adventures. I had done a lot of swimming as part of my fitness training. It felt ridiculous that now I could barely move in the water, and that with the aid of floats on both arms. I had a visit from a training buddy at the pool during one session and the pathetic nature of the sight of my bald nut and frail frame bobbing around was mitigated by our mutual laughter at this ridiculous scene. I found it refreshing that all the aspects of maintaining the 'gym-guy' pose were gone, and that I could have a good laugh about the seeming irrelevance and stupidity of it in comparison to where I was now. My overriding thinking was that everyone was going to end up dying someday due to eventual bodily failure of one kind or another; I was just getting there a little sooner than most. I felt that I'd aged in my mind and fast-forwarded to an advanced age, contemplating death. Nothing to lose. Nothing to worry about. Pain was nothing new now. I knew that statistically, I was as good as dead anyway, and I felt relaxed about it, even serene. So here I was on my back in warm water, nothing to bother me, feeling no pain, nice and peaceful, floating away in my own personal oasis.

The routine of eating, sleeping and hydro was broken up by blood tests every few days to measure my 'markers'. An innocuous word until it was explained that these indicators could show how much of a particular protein was swanning around my veins, betraying the presence of tumour cells looking for a new home. It was as if my vascular system could sense when a needle was near and retreated away. Tourniquets and bowls of warm water being the only way to ensure enough of an appearance to give a viable amount for a testable sample.

The results were showing a declining number. The oncology department was achieving the desired result and it seemed as if the tumour had been shrunken to the point where its removal had succeeded, and there didn't seem to be many nasties still in circulation. I was gaining some encouragement from all of this but not enough to see any further into the future than the next appointment. I figured out that if I could just keep clocking up one after another, I was surviving one day, two, five days, a week and so on. It had still only been just over three months since the diagnosis, but that seemed like years ago now. I had grown up. Coming into hospital as a typically arrogant, young man and here I was, a newly-minted sage with accumulated wisdom that comes with adversity and a very real brush with eternity.

My former life as a musician had now totally receded; my Royal Academy days over, music career prospects annihilated. Thousands of hours of practice, rehearsals, performances, adrenaline ups and downs all defined somebody else.

*****

The next three chemo sessions ran from early March to the end of April 1986, following the usual routine – same reactions, more weight loss. I recall that I'd plummeted down to 11 stone from my usual 13 and a half. I felt insubstantial and took on the generic, anonymous cancer patient look. Occasionally, when travelling to and from hospital, I did receive the odd stare, and once in a while, 'Oi, where did you get that nut, where did you get that nut?' to the old music hall tune. This was in the days of resplendent 1980's hairstyling, so a bald person was either a skinhead or on chemo. The fact I hadn't had to shave in six months made me appear younger too. I found this quite amusing, knowing that the explanation of the cause of all this was enough to freeze the blood in the veins of anyone who heard the story. It's down to the burden of knowing that everything else, all the vanity of striving, will end in death one day and that everyone is terrified of the existential void, even if they have a mechanism to fill that gap. Death is death, after all. As the Bard said, no one's returned from there to tell us how it is in terms universally accepted as yet.

As a patient on treatment, I had gone into a kind of living limbo, the passing of time delineated by the changing of bags of drugs on the frame, injections, blood tests, X-rays, and always the punctuation of vomiting, loose bowls and the rest. I was in no way taking in enough food or drink to be producing this. It must be the actual substance of my body dissolving. It felt that way anyway.

A strong enough breeze could get me airborne, I was convinced.

My final chemo was started on 22nd April. I didn't know if it was to be the final one but according to the MRC trial protocol, it was the last throw of the dice for this particular treatment.

A soul-deep exhaustion had set in. I didn't care anymore, had no goals, expectations or forward thinking. What I did have deep, deep down in me somewhere was the single thought that as far as I could, I would not allow these circumstances to kill my spirit; the other place I could get to in my mind away from this reality usually aided and abetted by music. I mused as to whether the saying might be true – that which does not kill me makes me stronger – and if I might be able to prove that. And there it was

– I had a goal; simply to survive and if that happened, let all the rest figure itself out.

*****

It must have been days later on a bright, sunlit part of the sixth floor. I must have been out of it in a metoclopramide-induced sleep. I heard a very distant voice, male, deep, comforting, calling me.

'Fred, Fred. It's all over, Fred.' Slowly, as I started to come to, I realised that my hand was being held in the strong grip of a rough and calloused hand, the hand of a working man. I put it all together; the resonant voice telling me it's all over, the feel of a strong working man's hand, maybe the hand of... the Carpenter from Nazareth! For a long time, I didn't dare to open my eyes, yet felt that I should try because it was...

Actually, it was a mate of mine, Ronald the joiner, and not Jesus after all, and I was evidently still in Fulham Palace Road and not Heaven.

I explained that I thought he'd come to usher me through the great and pearly gates – we had a good laugh about that. I asked him about the choice of phrase and he said the nurses had explained I was on my sixth and last treatment.

We talked on and laughed some more, and I promptly crashed out again. When I came back around, Ronald had gone off and I noticed that the ward was empty. I felt somewhat lonely and played through my mind the faces of my recent ward-mates, particularly Jeff. I hoped he was doing well. He'd been let out before me to go on holiday. The members of staff had rotated so there was no one in who knew him. I also remembered our nurse, Margaret, who'd shown us both exemplary care and kindness, though I knew Jeff was rather keen on her. Maybe it was reciprocated. I missed them.

A little later, a young man, purposeful and bold, walked in. I assumed he was a Registrar. I was disabused of that notion when he plonked himself down on the opposite bed. Soon afterwards, a nurse came in and drew the curtains around his bed. Not a doctor at all, it seemed. A new patient, probably.

After some more sleep, I awoke to find myself free of drips and feeling comfortable enough to look around and see how my new companion was doing.

I never found out his name. He was busily engaged in some obvious work-related reading. I cast him as a typically young, thrusting executive-type, too busy to be sick.

'Hello mate. What are you in for then?' My standard in-hospital ice-breaker.

One word, 'Testicular' said it all. He looked down and carried on reading.

It was patently obvious that the sight of me represented everything this chap was terrified of coming his way, almost entirely the feeling I'd had on seeing the man in the bed opposite me, back when my treatment started. I really hope he made it.

＊＊＊＊＊

After eventual discharge, life became a round of follow-up appointments, weekly blood tests, frequent X-rays and a constant dread of any strange aches and pains that always grew into unimaginable horrors of more cancer.

It was a strange and unaccustomed time. Not being immersed in the processes of surgery and chemo, doctor's rounds and continual attention from nurses can create a great empty feeling of deflation. The big question of 'What next?' Was there going to be a next? Where and how do you pick up the old threads? A life fully circumscribed by the rigours of studying to be a musician, performing, writing, working and socialising completely broken open. The other big question: 'What's left?'

There must have been a rumour that I'd died as my mother told me she'd had few phone calls asking how it had been at the end. These days, people record the mind-numbing minutiae of their minute by minute existence online and broadcast everything to the world. Back then, it was possible to fall entirely off the radar, which had certainly happened to me in the music circles in which I had moved. Presumably, my parents had told the Royal Academy what had been going on and, two and two being put together, it must have been assumed that it wasn't likely I'd survive.

So, here I was, back home, nothing to do except sit and wait. The occasional walk around the block on crutches. Sleeping a lot between hospital visits. Waiting for the test results, always anticipating the call back in.

I vividly remember what I have come to call my 'day of self-pity'; sitting alone at home, completely bored, tired and worn. Everyone else's life was moving on, as I was hearing from a declining number of visitors. I had a few hours of dismal gloom, culminating in a proper, full-on shoulders heaving weeping session, complete with hyper-ventilation and so on. It was good to release that and get it out of my system. Not coming from a family that was particularly big on the expression of emotions, this was a needed response and I thoroughly relished the feelings of relief afterwards. It was a decent pain-killer too. I had declined the offer of a prescription of Omnopon, although it did seem appealing at the time to have oblivion on tap. I did not want to come to rely on it.

Taking stock of the situation was difficult but necessary. I was still the same person basically, but I had been taken on an unwelcome, unexpected journey by cancer. I surmised that the old drives that had helped me to achieve what I had done up to the point of diagnosis, combined with the fact that I was still alive, could work together and perhaps be a new start in some way.

Chapter Five

Ramble On

Music: *The Song Remains the Same - Led Zeppelin*

My parental home had once had six of us sharing the modest two-storey terrace. When we moved there in 1966, Fulham was nothing like the area it has since become. I had moved back in, and now it was my parents and I; my siblings having all moved away, were married, raising families. Here I was, nearly 25 years old and starting all over again, this time an only child. And it has to be said, I had the capabilities and capacities of a child after my recent experiences.

I had no place of study, no work – everything had reset itself. Not even a piano in the house anymore. It had been well over half a year since I'd even looked at a piano. In terms of keeping your technique in order, a layoff like that might as well be as many years (perhaps slight hyperbole). I had never been away from the instrument for anything approaching this length of time. No possibility of seeing if I still had 'it', and I was even wondering if I had the will to play anyway. Had I really been a performer? Who, where was that fearless bloke? He'd been killed off along with the lump, so it appeared. I didn't particularly want to hear any 'classical' music. Too much of a reminder. I wasn't reading either, didn't have any concentration. Couldn't keep the thread of anything that required memory. In fact, I wasn't at all interested in

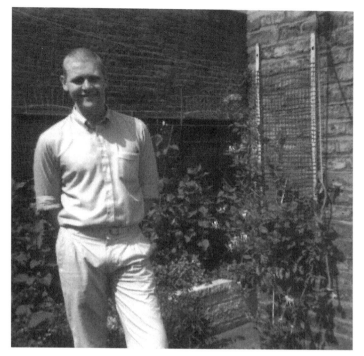

In recovery with hair growing back

anything much. I got out and about around the block on crutches now and again, still under orders to restrict contact with people, especially if they had the sniffles or any kind of communicable disease. My immune system was still shot to pieces.

Little by little, the fine, stubbly hair growth on my head began to manifest in blond, baby-hair curls, much to my mother's delight. To me, it further exemplified the return to earlier years. The blood tests were still favourable so it was looking like the cancer cells were either wiped out or at the very least dormant. So I began to see hair growth as a positive. I was told at an outpatient appointment that after your hair follicles are obliterated, it is often the case that you grow back a more lustrous covering in any case.

It was around this time that an event occurred that was to have deep significance to me and my later life. A professional musician friend called Roy came to visit and said he had something for me. Expecting food or similar, I was extremely surprised when he came back with a large flight case. Opening it up, he explained that he thought I might appreciate some music. The case contained a Yamaha DX7 synthesiser. Back in the 1980s, the DX7 was a ground-breaking, new technology in the music industry, a frequency modulation keyboard with its distinctive, unmistakable and characteristic sound. Just about every artist of the R 'n' B persuasion was using that FM sound. And so here I was, sitting on the floor of our front room with a DX7 hooked up to a small amp. I doubt if Roy had an idea of the power of that gesture all those years ago. After a bit of banter, he left and said I could hold on to the keyboard as long as I needed it.

At first, I had no idea what to do, what to play, and I was remarkably coy about it, keeping the volume as low as possible in marked contrast to the days when I was serially banished from practice rooms due to the length and volume of my piano practice sessions. Eventually, after a bit of skillful negotiation and donation, I had a piano housed in a local church where I could come and go and play to the big empty building as much as I wanted. And I often did, starting sometimes as early as 4.30a.m. in my keenness and drive to excel. I had a special set of counterweights installed in the action of the Bechstein grand I was using, which made the action particularly heavy to play. A bit like wearing wrist weights to play tennis, I suppose. The net result was I had developed considerable finger dexterity and strength, and a slight tendency to the heavy-handed, it has to be said. I appreciated the forbearance of the Vicar, who had said to me one day that he very much enjoyed my playing, but mentioned that my sound had a very penetrating property, especially at five in the morning. And now I was scared to make any kind of sound. I remember exactly what I played; it is engraved on my memory. Music is an incredibly powerful part of life. It is *the* universal language of expression in any culture or environment. When words have failed, music articulates pure emotion. The few notes and chords I managed to play seemed like the effort of someone stumbling around in a dark place, bearing no relation to what I used to be able to do.

*****

By way of a bit of background about my relationship to music, I was rather a late starter and came to music accidentally near the age of 14, the circumstances around which may have supplied the necessary determination that helped me progress rapidly.

I had started off quite well in the transition to grammar school and was near the top of the class for the first couple of years. I then made some ill-advised alliances and consequently found myself in significant trouble for my several misdemeanours. It was put to me that I had two alternatives; continue in the vein I had been accustomed to and face the inevitable correction, or completely turn the situation around, distance myself from previous associations and stay out of trouble. This all happened around the time of the screening of the TV drama, *Scum*, on the BBC. My future was graphically described to my parents and me by the relevant authorities. The reaction during that meeting of my parents was the motivation for me to more fully appreciate where this could go and the effect on them. They must have said many things in my defence that I was not party to, but sufficient to allow me a second chance subject to staying out of any further unfortunate situations.

Duly enlightened, I realised how serious this had been and could turn out to be if I didn't change. The conditions were that I would need to stay away from certain acquaintances, and be either at school or at home, according to a strict timetable. Any deviation would have consequences, and if at any point my parents found me uncooperative or impossible to handle, I would find myself living in a place I wouldn't choose to.

I knew I had broken the hearts of my parents. They had put themselves out for me, stuck up for me, and had been instrumental too in securing the current arrangement. I owed it to them to try.

At this time, my father experienced a serious recurrence of Crohn's disease, which had been more or less the pattern of his life from his mid-20s, when treatments were primitive. He endured an incredible amount of suffering but was always a model of stoic courage and strength. The thought went through my mind that I had caused this relapse, and this added to my determination to start again.

Life was extremely boring at this time, and so it was with some sense of relief that an old, decrepit upright piano appeared in our living room. I seem to recall it had been given to us as an interesting piece of furniture. That John Spencer upright with the dodgy keys turned out to be my salvation. I had always listened to music and so to alleviate the crushing boredom, discovered that I could find the right notes to many of my favourite songs. At that time, I was particularly keen on what is now termed 'prog rock'; Emerson Lake and Palmer, Yes, Pink Floyd, to name a few. I had worked up a version of the *Hallelujah Chorus* in an arrangement Rick Wakeman had incorporated into another song. I had seen the film *Rollerball*, the epic, dystopian vision of Norman Jewison, which opened with a dark screen to the sound of Bach's eerily powerful *Toccata* in D minor. I figured out my own way of playing this one too.

Around this time, my father had several visits from a district nurse, Eira Rowley. She happened to hear me playing one day and asked if I was having lessons. My first thought was to deliver a mouthful of outrage and indignation. Was she insane? Did she seriously think I was some kind of weird hermit with no friends? Back then, even though I enjoyed listening to music, my opinion of boys at school who played an instrument was that they were odd, lonely losers who had no real relationship to the outside world. I kept this to myself. Eira went on to explain that her own children were having lessons with a lady in Hurlingham. And this was how I came into contact with the most significant person, other than my parents, in my life up to that time – Florence Creighton, pianoforte teacher. This remarkable, patient, inspiring and demanding mentor, did she but know it at the time, saved my life and my future by kindling in me and eventually bringing to extraordinary fruition a love and devotion to music that came to dominate and inform my life.

Three years after that first meeting with Mrs Creighton, I was admitted to the Royal Academy of Music in London, where I remained a student up to the time of my diagnosis. As a result of being Mrs Creighton's student, I took my ABRSM grade exams at her house. One of my examiners happened to be the eminent British composer, Justin Connolly. Apparently, he was curious as to my progress and ability after Mrs Creighton had told him I was a late starter and that I also composed music. Justin agreed to take me on for composition lessons, after he had completed a piece to deadline for the Proms at the Royal Albert Hall. This was the start of a firm friendship that persists to this day.

However, all of that seemed to have passed me by. Any aspirations I'd had were gone. All I had was the memory of having been a pianist and composer. I could remember places I'd played, big concerts, exciting times, but these receded into what had become history to me. The cancer treatments had somehow put years on me and stolen the part of my identity defined by those musical achievements.

*****

Roy's generous act of kindness lit a small fire somewhere. Not long after dropping the keyboard at my house, he asked if I was up to attending a jam with some friends of his. Feeling completely out of my depth, I agreed, despite all my feelings of total technical inadequacy.

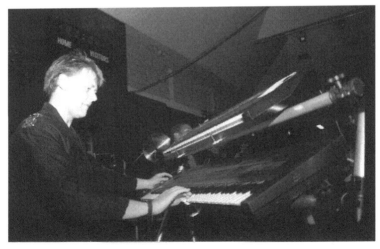

Working again thanks to Roy

I learned an extremely valuable lesson here. If someone has completely lost their way, it is often the case that the faith of someone who acts out of nothing but true altruism towards that person can bring them back from a dire situation. That was now my own experience on a number of occasions; having felt that cancer was nearly successful in wiping me out, several people independently had profound influence over the future course of events. Whether it was the well-meaning question of a district nurse showing an interest, the benevolence of a piano teacher, the kindness of a composer, a surgeon's skill, a friend's faith, all these conspired together to change the fortunes of an aimless survivor. When you give to someone who has nothing to give back to you, and for no possible advantage to you, the giver, you are showing the greatness of what true human compassion can do.

Anyway, this jam session was to be my re-introduction to the world of music making. Apart from being one of the original members of the 80's disco super-group *Heatwave*, Roy ran a highly-sought-after music production company that provided essential services to the major TV shows of the day, including *Top of the Pops*. Roy arranged for me to be his session keyboard player. This was a significant departure from the realms of the highbrow classical genre, requiring the ability to adapt to any and every style, learn a new song in a heartbeat, move it to any key for the benefit of the vocalists, and be proficient in a 'one-take' sense. As always in the music business, time was money, and so record companies appreciated work done quickly and accurately. I discovered that I was good at this and so we had a successful collaboration on many projects. Having earned a measure of credibility in this way, I came to the attention, through Roy, of his bandmates in *Heatwave* and ended up playing with the band in Europe and the US. The music and arrangements of their great classic dance tunes, *Boogie Nights*, *Always and Forever* etc. are etched in my mind and fingers to this day. Bopping around behind a keyboard A-frame rig was a great way to keep up the necessary discipline of physio on my knee replacement and associated muscles.

The greatest part of all this was that I had re-engaged with people through music and was active again, albeit in a different direction.

At one of our rehearsals in a studio in Amelia Street, near the salubrious surroundings of Elephant and Castle, I was busy sorting out the settings on my keyboard rig when a very confident and very beautiful, young lady – one of the backing singers – approached me and asked me something about the keyboards. I recognised her as a friend of Melanie's but her forthrightness was unusual. As a full-fledged moody muso, and not used to this kind of interaction, my response was both stupid and arrogant,

'You've seen keyboards before...? Well... it's like that.'

I certainly did not imagine that our paths would cross a few years later in a much more significant way.

I found myself from time to time in the presence of a piano. Not much inclined towards that instrument, it took a while before I felt like approaching one. In the unlikely surroundings of the sedate seaside town of Herne Bay was a farm converted into a record company recording facility. Between rehearsals, I noticed a Steinway grand and found myself alone with this magnificent beast during some downtime. With some trepidation, I took my place at the instrument, thought hard about a fitting piece to play, and summoned up the opening gestures of Beethoven's *Sonata Op. 111 in C minor*, the great Ludwig Van's final utterance in this form for piano. The great German pianist, Wilhelm Kempff, wrote that this opening is like two hands fashioning a great arena, the site of an upcoming colossal struggle. The image was not lost on me as I realised that my piano technique had largely evaporated. If I were to regain the ability to do what I had been able to before, it would undoubtedly be a battle. Something in me relished the prospect.

Chapter Six

Love of My Life

Music: *Through the Fire – Chaka Khan*

Having been brought up in a large family with four siblings, and having witnessed the inexorable growth of their extended families, it had not escaped my notice that I was probably never going to be in their situation, due in the first instance to the presumed long-term effects of chemotherapy then my disastrous prognosis, and last but not least, the absolute undesirability of me as a life partner for anyone, due to my comprehensively poor medical history. Who would want to be with a newly-disabled cancer victim?

On the music side, things were going from strength to strength, and I discovered through necessity, trial and error that I had the requisite skills to be a reliable session musician. Turn up on time, don't talk to the principal artist, be flexible, do what the producer asks and preferably on the first take. I learned the invaluable attribute of being sociable and easy to get along with. Combined with punctuality and sensitivity to the prevailing dress code, this will propel anyone forward in life. It was around this time too that my own music was beginning to attract some serious attention. Through the influence of British composer Michael Finnissy, a work of mine, *Boole* (for piano and nine instruments, written as a commemoration of the work of Irish mathematician George

Boole, of symbolic logic fame) was scheduled for performance at the Huddersfield Contemporary Music Festival. This serves as a showcase for new music, some might say avant-garde or related epithets. Gratefully and somewhat nervously, I took my seat at the concert. As the performers assembled on stage and tuned up, I heard a conversation between two fellows in the row directly behind me.

One of them said, 'I've come to hear that piece by Scott.'

'Oh, did you know him?'

'Yes, he was at the Academy, did quite a few concerts. Busoni, modern stuff mainly. Interesting.'

'What's he doing now? I haven't heard much.'

'Well you wouldn't. He died. Cancer, I think it was.'

Before a response could come, the music began. My mind was racing during the whole thing. Imagine the surprise when during the applause, I turned and greeted my friends. We went off for a couple of beers and a game of pool, as you would.

Nonetheless, despite once more having a viable music career, I couldn't help but feel alone. A cancer patient's life is lived in the spaces between appointments for tests, which at any time can reveal unwelcome news. It was as if an invisible umbilicus connected me to Charing Cross oncology department, always pulling me back.

One particular set of tests was concerning; I was seeing a registrar for follow-up and he looked intently at the usually routine chest X-ray, with the obligatory chin-stroke and pursed lips of concentration. Then, eye contact.

'Hmm. Well Mr Scott...'

'It's Fred. So why are you looking at that for so long?' I shouldn't have asked. A rare violation of my policy of disinterest.

'It's the shadow in your left lung, there, can you see it?'

Yes, I could see it, a big, brooding, dark patch.

'And?' I kind of knew what was coming next.

'Your cancer might have spread to the lung, that's the shadow, there.'

I must stress that the young doctor's candour was unusual; the more senior consultants had always been more circumspect. I could scarcely believe that this chap was going to have the final, authoritative say in this matter.

'In any case, I would need to get another view on this,' and with that comforting thought, he went off, presumably to find a colleague.

Upon his return, and after I'd had more than enough of looking at this particular X-ray, he said, 'Well, it's the weekend and since nobody's around, can you come back on Monday and we'll get someone else to look at it?' Rhetorical or not, this question, I agreed.

What a fabulous weekend ahead, full of visions of slow, painful death, amidst more horrible treatments. Perhaps they'd not try to treat this. If it's spread to the lungs, that's surely it? All these thoughts and more occupied me over that weekend. Very disappointing. Just when everything was picking up, it was all about to get rolled up. The clock seemed to spin rather than tick and soon enough, I was back at oncology, waiting for confirmation of the news. I had checked in and gave the receptionist my name, thinking you have no idea that they're about to tell me that I now have cancer in my lung, do you? Waiting rooms of oncology departments can be very difficult places to experience. People looking fully fit, yet anxious. Could be a relative waiting for someone or a new patient showing up for the first time. Others were in wheelchairs, hooked up to drips. Still others, thin, bald, barely visible, exuding hopelessness.

My turn, after an interminable wait.

'Fred, how are you?'

I had lined up a few responses, mostly sarcastic, but they didn't come out. I was silent, grimly stoic.

'Well, we've looked at the film and that shadow...' here it comes... 'is a fault with the print. There's nothing there actually.'

I felt that I'd escaped, been released, smiled upon. This experience formed in me the attitude that no matter what I was told, in terms of bad news, I was not obliged to accept it as the only truth. Over that weekend, and indeed since diagnosis, I had never actually wanted to die. Accepting the possibility yet not really willing to surrender to the idea. Since being discharged after the final chemo session, I was a very frequent visitor to Charing Cross for follow-up tests, as I've said. Life increasingly became defined as the reprieve after each review. Life was lived in initial units of days, then weeks, and later months between tests. To this day, I don't think it's been longer than six months at a stretch when I've not been called in for follow-up tests. Cancer is a constant companion, the all-unwelcome guest everywhere I am always. At that point, even though I had resumed a career in music, life was all about the devastation of cancer. Every step was a reminder of being held up by an artificial knee joint. Every pain a potential problem. As I began to travel, every airport security gate, a long story to an incredulous official. Even though I always carried a small copy of an X-ray of my knee, I always had to explain the odd-looking metal object and have my leg squeezed or prodded. During those heightened times of security, I was routinely separated from travelling companions in order to explain myself. At a checkpoint in an Asian airport stopover, and because I was not in command of the language, the X-ray seemed to arouse some unwanted excitement. A clearly agitated military person with an imposing gun was evidently unimpressed. The universal language of aggression and demand communicated clearly that unless I could sort this out, I wouldn't be going anywhere. So with an open-handed gesture of conciliation and an imploring look, fighting a sense of outrage in the realisation that I couldn't talk this chap down, I started to undo my belt, other hand still in the air, and slowly loosened my trousers. He'd either think this was a colossal insult or that I was slightly insane. Graciously, he waited until I had dropped my strides to reveal the massive scar. Pointing to this and the X-ray made the desired impact. He lowered the gun, smiled and waved me on. I had now been humiliated internationally, and despite a strong urge to express in no uncertain terms how I didn't deserve this, I walked off to join my fellows.

'Get that a lot, do you?'

'Every time. Must be my aftershave.' Well, who else can say they'd mooned an armed security official and walked away to tell the tale? Truly, cancer opens doors closed to most others.

Opening doors and all the attendant excitements apart, and despite being back in music, my life was still a seemingly ceaseless round of check-ups. The ebb and flow of tension and relief between these hospital visits provided a kind of exhilaration, the systole and diastole of condemnation and reprieve.

So this was to be it; a musician of sorts after all, playing and recording love songs for nobody in particular until it was all ended anyway by resurgent cancer cells.

In the midst of this scenario, I got to know my future wife. Against all the odds and expectations, we are together, having celebrated our 25th anniversary at the time of writing, with our three children. When I was in the midst of chemo, I never entertained the fantasy of having a family, assuming it wouldn't happen. Even when we were newly married, we never assumed there would be a chance of a family, but importantly, neither we did we assume the opposite. We were just happy to be together, in love.

Not wanting to gloss over this period of time in one sweep, this proved to me that, as the ancient king/poet once said, 'love is stronger than death', or in our case, the regular threat that it would all be over much too soon.

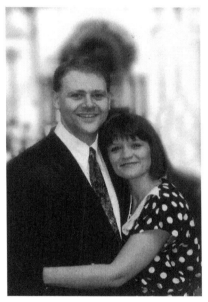

Newlyweds 1990

Interestingly, this is the traditional point where, in a fairy tale, everyone lives happily after, end of story. The reality for a cancer survivor and anyone associated with or even married to one is that the whole complex of forces around survival and outcomes looms large. Cancer rarely just packs up and goes. Its legacy takes many forms, some physical, others less tangible, more subtle. We had opened the door on a life, never dull, yet full of uncertainty, from day one. Add into that mix the children and the whole thing becomes surreal.

Our children have always lived with the challenges that my situation placed on the family. We have never made a particularly big deal of all the ins and outs of cancer and its impact.

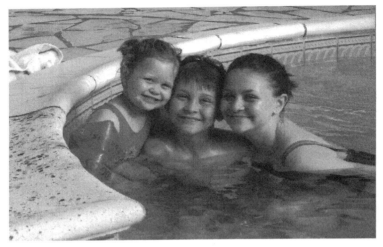

Family holiday 2007

If that fateful, mercifully false X-ray had been an authentic harbinger of death then so be it. There would be little in the way of consequences outside myself. I was now supporting a family. The mind is focussed on such things as making sure you stay healthy, even though that's only partly under your control. I reflected often that I had contracted cancer whilst being young, fit, strong, ambitious and totally healthy, for no apparent reason, perhaps best explained by Shakespeare's Edmund in *King Lear*: 'We make guilty of our disasters the sun, the moon and the stars.'

We loved each other and resolved simply to get on with life and take it as it presented itself on a daily basis. As I said, that was about 25 years ago. Nothing's changed. The tale of those intervening years is what follows.

Chapter Seven

'We Can Revise Him'

Music: *Carl Nielsen, Symphony No. 4 'Det Uudslukkelige'*

Since it's not my intention to populate this account with details of our family life, my focus is on the legacy and daily realities of living under the shadow of cancer. By now, and at the age of 54, I have lived more of my life as a cancer survivor than otherwise by a couple of years, to no one's greater surprise than my own. The gift of my family remains an incomprehensible blessing and daily source of wonder; a perfect antidote to the self-focus that can inevitably come with serious illness. In my experience, your life can be defined by what you choose to allow it to be. Whilst it is true that cancer is a relentless, insidious presence once it's touched you, the choice is there to give up on living or wring out of each minute you have, every drop of life, not knowing how many minutes are left. In our risk-averse society, we like to believe we have every contingency covered, planned out, certain of the outcome. In reality, nothing is further from the truth. For most, our existence is controlled by fear and too easily, the sovereign spark of life and its possibilities are swallowed up in anxiety. There is enough happening in the world sometimes to convince us that everything is against us.

This background chatter is unlikely to go away as it is undoubtedly part of our intrinsic humanness, the innate defence mechanism that has allowed our survival through evolutionary rigours, and I am not saying it's a bad thing – far from it – but surely we can allow ourselves a look upwards and forwards as well.

Cancer is both a death sentence and a life sentence. More than most, you are brought into the closest proximity with your end but not knowing specifically when that will be. However, all human life will end in bodily death under whatever circumstances. No one can be sure about the timing; it's just that cancer makes you face the probability in an intimate way.

*****

There was always uncertainty as to how long my artificial knee and femur would last given the exigencies of wear and tear, mechanical failure, cancer recurrence and a host of other imponderables (certainly, I had no desire to ponder them). Such operations are not usually done on the young. A replacement means your limb is spared in the first instance and the disease hopefully excised. What happens later though, when the metal ages?

To entertain this question presupposes that you will survive the cancer long enough to actually need this even to be a consideration.

We had been fortunate enough to travel quite a bit for work and live abroad for a while, and after a period of several years, I had managed to get back into a regular fitness programme involving a lot of swimming, making sure my children were strong swimmers too. Contact sport, running, racket sports et al. had been ruled out on account of the effects of impact on what was left of my leg and the metal. However, after several years, the joint began to behave slightly erratically – my gait changed; I developed a tendency for my left foot to kick out at a rather more pronounced angle. Increasing pain in the thigh alerted me to the need for a serious consultation. Whenever I had a doctor's appointment abroad, my case was always met with incredulity.

'How on earth did you survive that?' was a common question, together with, 'And why did you have a knee replacement so young?'

It was now about 14 years after the initial operation and during a visit to Mr Anthony Hall, now at Chelsea and Westminster Hospital, it was decided that I'd had a good run (excuse the irony) with this joint, and surprising longevity, which I attribute to Mr Hall's genius, and that it was time to do something about it. I had always made the assumption from day one, back in 1985, that if I did not die immediately, I would probably succumb to cancer of one form or another before the issue of joint wear and tear came up. There was also the burgeoning feeling that this situation could and would have a serious impact beyond me; there was my family to consider. Anything that was about to happen to me was also about to happen to us, my wife and, at that time, two young children. The idea of the lone patient soldiering on alone didn't work now. I was the head of a family unit with responsibilities beyond simply being cheerfully philosophical.

My first thought was this; metal doesn't regenerate, obviously. I didn't need a medical degree to figure that out. Was straight amputation on the cards? I'd delayed it for over a decade after all. Maybe they could fix the thing in a splint so that I wouldn't be able to bend it; a straight leg is better than no leg, surely?

After all, there's nothing wrong with my foot!

For the first time, I heard the name of Mr Steve Cannon, Consultant Orthopaedic Surgeon and specialist in the art and science of knee revisions. This is the operation to replace a previous knee replacement. Mr Hall said that his colleague was the top man in this field and with that assurance, I was introduced to a hospital I'd vaguely heard of – the Royal National Orthopaedic Hospital, Stanmore. This is a place with a long history of clinical excellence in complex procedures. RNOH is recognised as a world centre for difficult orthopaedic surgeries of all kinds. In my mind, this at least offered the possibility of keeping my leg. Surely Mr Hall would not have referred me if he was unsure of the outcome?

I began to imagine how on earth you remove a prosthesis cemented into your bones, embedded in your tissues for nearly a decade and a half! Not being much given to metalwork or engineering, I declined further speculation and decided to see how Mr Cannon proposed to manage this feat.

The first impression of a visit to RNOH, Stanmore is that you've come to the wrong place. Surely this rather random collection of Second World War pre-fab huts is a relic of that great conflagration; an army training camp, perhaps? Certainly a museum piece and surely not a working hospital?

Sadly, the truth remains that this great and irreplaceable institution is housed in the most ramshackle accommodations imaginable in the 21st century for the kind of work that is done there. At the time of writing, there is an ongoing appeal for funds to re-build the site. If you have persevered with reading this far, please reward yourself by making a donation to the RNOH charity.

Meeting Mr Cannon was not unlike my first encounter with Mr Hall, with the exception that I was not lying down this time. He exuded the same kind of quiet authority, registrars hanging on every word, scribbling notes attentively.

Mr Cannon was evidently surprised that the prosthesis had lasted as long as it had. I was wondering if this was a preamble, lining me up for some consolation before the inevitable recommendation of amputation. I was in turn surprised when he suggested that a revision would be viable in my case, with the caveat that if the circumstances he discovered during surgery were too adverse then I might very well wake up minus the limb. A visitor to the outpatient department at Stanmore will never fail to see evidence of the extremity of the conditions that are treated there. RNOH started life as a children's hospital and has dedicated units for these surgeries. The fact that a child can leave the place able to stand straight and walk tall again is nothing short of miraculous. Being in the waiting room is a salutary experience. There is usually a mix of cancer patients, as at Charing Cross, but also extreme cases of conditions obviously requiring complex intervention. It's hard to be there and not be profoundly moved.

I have never taken good health for granted since my own cancer diagnosis, but rather resolved to do what I can in whatever way I can to raise awareness and funds for this great place.

Sitting on my hospital bed after admission, I realised that my 'good run' had come to an end. Meetings with the surgical team and pre-op tests done, I now had time to contemplate where I was and what I was facing. This time, the crucial difference was that I was not the only one facing things; my wife and two children were at home, a long way away on the other side of London. There is a terrible ache in the heart to think of the impact of your health problems on your immediate family. My children had never known me as anything but their active, fit dad, out and about doing things together in the outdoors whenever possible, walking along with them on my shoulders, always plenty going on.

If this operation didn't go as planned, that life would be over for all of us.

Thoughts like this can become morbid and drag the spirit way down. This appeared to me to be selfish in the extreme. Surely the thing was to focus on getting out, getting better in whatever shape I was in; it would be enough to be alive and starting from there, do the best I could. As I had back in Charing Cross, I had carefully selected music with me on CD. The particular favourite this time round was the *Fourth Symphony* of Carl Nielsen, with the portentous sub-title, *Inextinguishable*. Evidently, it was the composer's wish to 'express what we understand by the spirit of life'. This was not lost on me as I saturated my mind with this fine, powerful masterpiece.

*****

Despite some understandable trepidation, the surgery went very smoothly and I came round in recovery, able to establish that my left leg was still there, as indicated by the severe but only too welcome pain.

The next several days were given over to some intensive physio and I was up on crutches within four days. As things had clearly moved on since Charing Cross, or maybe because I wasn't having chemotherapy this time, I was scheduled to go home on the fifth day.

We lived about a three-hour drive from Stanmore and although I felt every bump in the road, it was a relief beyond description to arrive home and walk, albeit with assistance, through the door that afternoon. I was envisaging continued physio, copious amounts of food and I'd be back to full strength in no time.

Evening came around and I felt exhausted, clearly the various substances I'd received just a few days previously and the various painkillers I had taken were still sloshing around in my system. I was sure I'd sleep well that night back with my family.

To the soundtrack of the mundanely domestic, I dropped off, smiling.

If you have ever seen that most notoriously gruesome tableau in the film *The Godfather*, involving a certain fictional film director, you will be able to visualise what happened next.

I became conscious bit by bit and was increasingly aware of dampness around me. I'd known this humiliation before back in Charing Cross during chemo. It was true I'd had an epidural as part of the anaesthesia and maybe the short term after-effects were a certain lack of functional control from the waist down, as it were. At least this was my waking thought. Mustering the strength to push myself up to a sitting posture, I swung the covers away to reveal a crimson pool spreading around me. There was no horse's head causing this. With growing incredulity and alarm, I realised that my lengthy scar must have split open, saturating the bed with blood. Unlike in the film, there was no cut-away to a presciently world-weary Don. This was real.

I called my wife in to see this and both of us, very calmly as it turned out, made a series of decisions. First was to take me as soon as possible to the nearest A & E department in South London. Around 11p.m., any London A & E on a Friday night was likely to be a very colourful place, beginning to be filled up by people the worse for wear after heavy drinking, fights and the like. I still wonder at her completely unfazed demeanour and inner reserves of strength facing what was happening to me, or rather to us.

After calling an ambulance we decided to secure the wound as best we could with as much sterile gauze as we could find in an ancient first-aid kit, wrapping the leg tightly in as much of that as we had then some bandage and finally, a bathroom towel.

Fortunately for a Friday night in London, we didn't have too long of a wait. After logging in at reception, I was wheeled into the department, which was full of patients, staff, security guards and police. Apparently, someone who had been brought in was violently threatening anyone who approached him.

I was deposited on a bed and left in a corridor. Figuring that I might be here for a while and concerned about what was going on under the makeshift wrappings around my leg, I attracted the attention of a passer-by and asked them to find a nurse. Pleading urgency, a nurse indeed came and at my request, wheeled me to the nearest phone from which I made a call to RNOH Stanmore. They insisted I come back up to them immediately. This was a serious relief and we were soon enough on the way back up to North West London. My wife had somehow managed to arrange a lift up to Stanmore.

An early-hours' drive up through busy Central London brought me back to the ward I had departed from only a few hours earlier.

A de-brief from the duty nurse and here I was as if I'd never left. The downside of being admitted on a Friday night/Saturday morning is that none of the consultants involved in my case were going to be around until Monday.

The characteristically expert re-dressing of the open wound reassured me I'd be all right until a proper assessment could be made by the surgical team. It appeared that the bleeding had been copious but had now stopped. All sorts of wild speculations coursed through my mind; I probably wasn't going to bleed to death but would they just cut it off now? Exhausted, I put on my headphones, (my wife had had the presence of mind under circumstances to pack my CDs) and let Bach take me off as Friedrich Gulda started the first *Prelude and Fugue* from the *Well-Tempered Clavier*.

It was a quiet weekend. No doctors rounds, no operations, just the routines of food, medications and catching up with the ward-mates I didn't think I'd see again. A new chap was in the bed opposite, a particularly friendly ex-soldier, Jason, who'd had an appalling accident on a motorbike, having survived active duty in the Gulf War and we struck up an immediate rapport. He'd arrived almost as soon as I had left.

It was disappointing to be here again, on the same day as being discharged. As Pacino's character said in a certain film not unrelated to one previously cited, 'Just when I thought I was out, they pull me back in.' I was certainly anxious to see Mr Cannon and figure out what on earth had gone wrong and where we needed to go from here. The one thing I knew was that I was in the right place.

The complexity and risk associated with revision surgery was coming home to me in a big way; signing a consent form with nonchalance one day, questioning everything the next. I was back in the hands of the doctors. Their decisions and actions were the crucial next steps.

Mr Cannon explained that I'd had a haematoma around the site of the operation – a collection of blood around the traumatised tissues – and there were many of those. I would need an immediate debridement; a procedure to investigate then wash out the area, under general anaesthetic. It was hoped that the viability of the initial operation could be preserved.

No stranger to the pre-operative phase, I wasn't bothered about a day-long fast. My surgery was an emergency and not on the schedule so I was to wait for all the others to be done before I went down to theatre.

'Oh dear, your veins are terrible,' said the anaesthetist. Many attempts to find an available entry point failed. 'I don't know if we'll be able to do this.' Given that we were in the ante-room to the theatre, and I could see the team gowned up, masked and ready, I realised that it was going to go ahead no matter what.

The thought occurred to me that it would be vastly preferable to be completely unconscious for this business but how was that going to be possible if they couldn't get the right juice into the right veins?

'Just breathe in as deeply as you can as I put this mask on you, it's gas and it should…'

And it did.

Coming round in the recovery room was every bit as uncomfortable as it had been the week before, again indicating that my leg was still there, and after the usual post-op vomiting had stopped and I could tolerate a few sips of water, the nurse and porter took me back to the ward.

'Don't try and move your head, Fred, please.'

What had they done to my head?

'It's just that the only place they could find for insertion of the anaesthetic was your neck. You've got a cannula there. Do try and keep still though. We'll take it out later.'

This was a new one on me. I became aware of a dull ache in my neck and an almost unbearable urge to turn my head round, just to stretch. When you're told not to do something, it's about all you can think of doing. In hospital, these things can become an obsession. All this lying around, trying to keep still inevitably meant that it wasn't long before I had to use my special manoeuvre, now well-practiced, to avoid the catheter. I was truly feeling back at square one. Hooked up, helpless and hospitalised. Regular exchanges of banter with Jason kept all this in perspective. Nielsen's symphony, Gulda's magnificent Bach, and a new release of Medtner piano sonatas from Marc-Andre Hamelin were enough to keep my mind active through the physical stasis and waiting around for a medical opinion on how things were going.

My leg was in a very delicate state; any movement I had gained from the previous operation was no longer there and I had to keep as immobile as possible to reduce further risk of haematoma. I had, perhaps fondly, thought that since I'd had a few good years after the chemo and first operation that it would be all easy from now on. Then I received some interesting news.

It appeared that a blood test was showing a rather high level of C-reactive protein (CRP). This indicated the presence of infection. A risk in all orthopaedic procedures, I had always been told that this was bad news. If it didn't settle down, the newly-installed metalwork would have to come out. The implications of this were alarming. After all, there's only so many of these operations a body can tolerate. I was now on my second replacement and if this one was infected... well, it didn't bear thinking about. It was 'wait and see'.

My friend, Jason, was scheduled for his surgery. We joked about how he'd survived a war and yet had been flattened in a bike accident locally to his West-Country home. Presumably, it would be a quick and relatively routine repair job.

Amid the usual chorus of well-wishing when someone's taken down to theatre, Jason was wheeled away on his bed. On and off during my usual cycle of analgesia-enhanced dozing, I noticed that it was taking a while for him to come back. As it turned out, we didn't see him back on the ward for a couple of days.

Apparently, there'd been a crisis during his operation. The long and short of it was that the drugs administered to him had reacted badly with whatever was in his system from his military days. Thankfully, after being returned to us, he told us of a nightmare landscape he'd found himself in; an infinitely large army of jelly babies in camo-gear crawling all over him had been one of the more humorous hallucinatory scenarios – funny yet terrifying.

A visit from Mr Cannon clarified what was happening with me. The large sleeve around my leg connected to a pump circulating cold water was to reduce the temperature and inflammation in the leg. It was proposed that I be put on some seriously strong antibiotics delivered intravenously. This was an unwelcome reminder of being back on chemo, with bags of fluid hung up next to the bed. A novel twist this time; the drugs would be delivered through four cannulas. Two were sited in the crook of each elbow, meaning I had to keep my arms straight, and two more were going into veins just above my ankles.

'Try and keep as still as you can, Fred. Don't want to disturb the flow,' said a cheerful, ruddy-cheeked registrar. Clearly a rugby-type. I'd observed that most orthopods in my experience were seriously strong types. Must be that the gentlemanly art of the oval ball prepares one for the physical conflagrations of the operating table.

I will not detain the reader with details of how this positioning of inflowing medicines through four cardinal points had an impact on my bodily routines, in particular feeding and elimination. Delicacy forbids I should elucidate.

In short, it took a further month to see a reduction of infection levels. During that time, my wife faithfully made an almost nightly journey across London, despite having to continue full-time work and the usual family responsibilities. It would have been impossible to conceive of going through all this without her. This was the incentive to get better, get out, and get home. Casually glancing at the television one morning, I caught sight of a programme my children enjoyed watching, *64 Zoo Lane*. Hearing the theme tune made me wail convulsively for them. It's a cliché but I simply had to get out of here for them, be strong and recover, however far from reality this appeared to be at that moment.

*****

During the ensuing weeks, the infection level remained stable and with no overt symptoms, it was decided that I should go home. If the infection were to be chronic, that is to say not going anywhere, it could theoretically be kept under control with antibiotics. I was to report any changes, flu-like episodes and the like, which would indicate that the bugs had gone systemic and action would need to be taken. Knowing that I was desperate to go home, I was prescribed some heavy-duty medicines and discharged.

It turned out I would be taking ciprofloxacin, a relatively new and powerful antibiotic, for most of the next decade. Apart from its use at the time as an anti-anthrax drug, I noticed some rather unpleasant side effects not yet listed in the *British National Formulary*, namely vividly terrifying hallucinatory nightmares. I suppose you can get used to anything, although it was always a great relief to wake up, which I usually did four or five times nightly.

I reflected that this had been my longest continuous stay in hospital and I had many sobering thoughts to contend with as I left RNOH, chief among them being the threat from this infection. I had learned that it is entirely possible for microbes to exist in a kind of 'bio-bubble' associated with the implanted metalwork and scar tissue surrounding the operation site. There had been considerable trauma from two procedures back to back. I wondered whether the prospect of rampaging infection was any worse than metastasising cancer cells; after all, both could kill you just as effectively. The real sting in all this was the effect on my wife and family, amplifying my concerns far beyond anything I had previously felt.

The metaphorical content of Nielsen's music was not lost in the midst of this – my physical body had sustained assaults from bone cancer, radical surgery and chronic infection. But the body is different from the mind, the spirit. I have a fundamentally optimistic frame of mind and despite the platitude, it is nevertheless true that adversity, if it doesn't kill you outright, can make you stronger. I had to live this out as if it were actually true. I had compelling reasons to stick with that attitude. I had certainly become sensitised to the triviality of many of our human concerns, and saw that most of these centre around fear of dying, physical pain and bad health. Looking out from this viewpoint gave me a very different, perhaps warped perspective; disease had warped my life so it was no wonder, after all. The use of 'gave' above is interesting and perhaps problematic. We hope to be given good things in life, but what happens if what you are given, along with the good, includes the appallingly bad? Why is it so common that we expect only good and fear anything other? Some might regard negative circumstances as a curse of some kind. The inevitable end of physical life is bodily death. The time it takes from birth to the unavoidable conclusion is open and unpredictable. Whole philosophies and religions have appeared as a response to the need to understand this fact. Without getting too metaphysical, at the time all this was going on, I resolved simply not to worry about what I could not alter and instead to be positive and love my family.

As Mr Cannon had said, 'We've done all we can.'

Chapter Eight
2001 – Beyond the Millennium

Music: *Ferruccio Busoni, 'Doktor Faust – Symphonia'*

Sixteen years since diagnosis. I had arrived at the year 2001.

I had just been old enough to witness the UK release of Stanley Kubrick's epic movie, *2001: A Space Odyssey*, which I saw at a large cinema near Tottenham Court Road with my dad when I was about eight or nine years old. This epic film is still considered enigmatic today, so little wonder it had such a profound impact on the mind of those of us of a certain age also witnessing the moon landing as a reality. The year 2000 as a concept had always fascinated people since the first digit revolves only once every thousand years.

What would the world be like in 2001? Would we routinely hop in and out of space, up to the moon, off to Jupiter, talk to computers and encounter alien intelligences?

Well, largely no, as it transpired. No one will argue that the biggest news of 2001 was not a mysterious object on the moon, but the events in New York on 11th September. It was a little after 2p.m. and I had the news on. I honestly thought that I was watching a disaster movie and not real life. I tried to call a friend in New York but all phone service to that city was out. It was a time of great unreality, uncertainty, surreal and world-changing. We were travelling quite a lot for various reasons and witnessed ever more heightening security and a pervasive feeling of threat and danger.

With two children now in primary school, we knew that we should travel less and needed to be around for them. One of our last long-haul trips had been to Australia to visit our best friends there. We'd been neighbours in fact and forged our friendships over much shared experience of child-rearing and the exchange of barbecuing techniques.

I was OK to travel as long as I had adequate supplies of antibiotics, and was generally cautious about health matters. One of my long-term prescriptions was for Ciproxin, which was useful against anthrax, and there had been a momentary disruption to my regular supply when it appeared in the news that certain suspicious white powders had been arriving in the mailboxes of prominent US and other politicians. As a precaution, Ciproxin had been stockpiled just in case. The fact I had it with me attracted attention, perhaps even more than my propensity to set off metal detectors with my prosthesis. Explanatory documents from my doctor usually did the trick.

Several hours into our flight to Australia, I was beginning to notice some significant discomfort below my left knee. It persisted and eventually I had to go and check it out after noticing a discharge making its way through my trouser leg. In the small aeroplane toilet, I made the grisly discovery that a section of skin under my knee joint's bend had reddened and was exuding a mixture of blood and white fluid. My shock was somewhat mitigated by knowing I had to pack this with tissue and put pressure on it. It was not so much flowing as slowly seeping through a small breach in the skin. I went back to my seat and related this latest development to my commendably calm wife. We decided to ask the cabin crew for whatever dressings they might have. There wasn't really much else to do at 30,000 feet. I was becoming progressively more uncomfortable and the pressure in my leg seemed to build. Despite our entreaties that I needed some space to stretch the limb out, we were advised that I had to stay where I was, that is to say standing up near the toilet. This went on for the several long remaining hours of the flight. As soon as we touched down, my friends took me straight to a medical centre. I contacted Stanmore and was advised to monitor what was happening while my consultant was contacted for advice. It turned out that I should stay where I was and hope that the situation stabilised. I should report back any major changes in 'output' or any flu-like symptoms – evidence of systemic infection building up. Our family visit to our good friends was now somewhat overshadowed by this development but we managed the situation and made the best of our time. I just had to keep taking the tablets, as it were, and change the dressings regularly.

Once back in the UK and up at Stanmore, we learned that the persistent peri-prosthetic infection was thriving in its comfortable environment and causing this reaction. The infection was essentially benign as long as it didn't pass around my body. This sounded rather reminiscent of what I'd been told about cancer cells back in the early days. So, the removal of the diseased bone and destruction of rogue cells by chemo had done its job back then. Now, the novel aspect of my revised metalwork was this infection. Apparently, we could coexist as long as I could put up with the consequent and seemingly endless exuding. However, it might just as quickly clear up as spontaneously as it manifested itself. I was getting more and more used to these kinds of uncertainties. My life had become one big uncertainty many years previously anyway. This was not new, just a major issue for my family. I did not want to drag them into all this. As I said before, love is stronger than death and the daily strength

I received from my family was without doubt the best medicine of all.

It wasn't long before a second breach appeared near the knee, and it too was now regularly exuding away. The option presented to me by Stanmore was for another operation to remove everything, clean out the area and try another revision. However, this might not work and I'd be just as vulnerable to infection as before due to the trauma and sheer amount of metalwork. We thought long and hard about the implications of all this. I decided to wait it out, not rush into another operation; I had a family to support. My children were growing up and that's an expensive time of life.

It's never a good idea to keep taking time off work, and employers that truly understand and are sympathetic to this fact of life for a cancer survivor are very rare. There is now much more general positivity to the idea that a greater number of people can expect to survive certain cancers. However, this means a correspondingly greater number of people needing to attend follow-up treatments and check-ups. How about employers responding to this with sensitivity rather than being forced to make token concessions by law? A cancer survivor is a tough, resourceful character with a serious perspective on life and not just damaged goods.

*****

It was around this time that I bumped into an old training buddy from my early gym days. We caught up on the passage of the last two decades, his life and times and my sudden departure from our circle. I will not forget his shock and the tears that followed a look at the damage to my leg. I interpreted these as sincere sympathy but assured him that I would not change a detail of my life if it meant that I'd not have my family. If my life so far had been leading up to where I was today in some or other kind of causal chain then it was all worth it. Every bit.

Our decision to travel less and some circumstantial changes gave us a more centred family life. I was doing more teaching and was based locally.

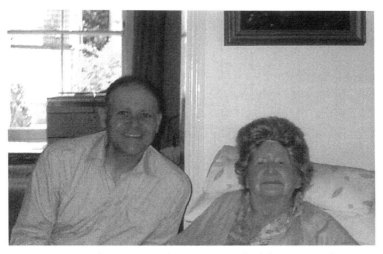

A visit to Florence Creighton, my wonderful piano teacher

Having our two children, now ten and seven was a daily joy. I never took this for granted due to the chemotherapy I'd had, and also just because of the sheer improbability of having made it as far as I had, now 20 years after diagnosis. Battered, bruised, leaking but still here.

After much discussion, we decided to try for another baby. It was a great delight when my wife became pregnant with our third child.

If the process of living had taken off a lot of my rougher edges then the birth of my second daughter turned me into an unashamedly blubbering softie.

However, my old adversary, cancer, may have been down but was by no means out. A term coined by Dr Philip Savage, my new Oncologist at Charing Cross, was 'sequelae'. My O-level Latin kicked in and I recognised this as a plural. Yes, cancer has sequels or, if you like, a legacy of subsequent effects. In my case, I had acquired a somewhat awkward gait, which had implications for certain muscular-skeletal functions. I was determined that I would be as careful, even as gentle, as possible with this revised knee and despite the infection, hoped that by such consideration, I wouldn't compromise it by anything I did. Life is unpredictable though and can be full of surprises.

One evening, I was attending to the mundane household chore of dealing with the kitchen after dinner. Getting the bin liner out of the pedal bin was always rather like assisting at the birth of some large, struggling pachyderm. I bent over to start the process and prepared to heft what I anticipated would be its usual not inconsiderable weight. The bin, however, being empty meant that I shot up quickly. Too quickly, and being fully braced for a heavy job, my momentum carried me further back beyond upright than I planned to go. Immediately, I was seized down the left side from lower back down to foot with searing, breathtaking pain. Pain that did not alter in intensity. Gasping, I called out to my wife. She could see I was in trouble and helped me somehow to inch into the bedroom, where I fell face down onto the bed. I was by now howling with this pain that wouldn't stop. As I was to learn the next day, this was sciatica, and I had seized a main nerve between vertebrae, the pressure ringing bells along my central nervous system. My wife called for a doctor and during an ensuing seemingly endless wait, normal painkillers being utterly useless, I resorted to the Discman. The CD already there was the Bach-Busoni *Chaconne*. I kept playing this over and over again, groaning along to its repeated theme and trying to focus only on its progression through ingenious variations. I became so grateful for this fabulous piece, I resolved to add it to my concert repertoire. When a locum visiting doctor eventually arrived, I tried to communicate that if he had anything in his bag that would knock over a horse or two then kindly get it into me as soon as possible by any means necessary. Despite a certain linguistic disconnect, I think my anguish communicated itself well enough. The impact of this new injury was that I now had quite serious numbness down the outside of my left leg and into my foot. Already essentially disabled by the previous surgery, I now had a lopsided hobble, supported by an old crutch we had kept.

It seemed that cancer, through a long and insidious process, had effectively and progressively disabled me.

*****

The chronic infection I had meant that I was applying up to four dressings to the site daily. My pharmacist was superb at suggesting combinations of materials that would help me make it through a working day without too much collateral damage to my clothing, although with even the best preparation, embarrassing patches on my leg were not that unfamiliar. The constant application of tape to secure the gauze patches in place led to a degradation of the skin, which began to be a concern. Eventually, another revision would be on the cards but the skin would have to be healthy enough to be able to heal. In other words, an operation could be successful, but compromised by the fact that the scar would not close up properly. Having had the incident of the haematoma, I didn't want another one. The sinus, to give it its technical name, was continually discharging and needed constant attention, dressing and cleaning to keep the skin viable for the future. It was hoped by both the doctors and me that the infection would eventually respond to the antibiotics or just spontaneously vanish. This did not happen. Instead, soon enough, another sinus appeared on the inside edge of the knee. Equal in output, this new sinus discharged regularly, necessitating two lots of dressings and cleaning up to four times a day. I considered this a small price to pay to keep my leg. It simply meant I had to look after quite a large area to ensure viability, and be careful about avoiding further infection to these new wounds. Having survived the initial cancer up to this point, I wouldn't want to be finished off by some rogue microbes.

I conducted a kind of health audit at that time; I was disabled, getting around on crutches, stooping due to the back injury, complicated by unpredictably painful sciatic jangling, and using an unprecedented number of dressings up to four times per day. To say this was onerous would understate the inconvenience, added to which I was working full-time to support my family and growing children through their secondary education. Being of a fundamentally optimistic frame of mind, and disposed in general to believing the best of people, I suppose I was surprised at how someone who is disabled can be treated by the uncomprehending. Obviously, there is a degree of sensitisation that accompanies being host to cancer cells and infections, inevitably affecting how you view others in a similar plight. Perhaps there is just a greater identification with the sufferings of others, but it has never failed to amaze me to what extent people unaffected by physical problems can view and act towards those of us who obviously are. I looked upon all this as an education in human nature. My conclusion is that if your own life is the actual fulfilment of the dreads of others in health terms, you become a walking 'memento mori' for them, which tends to intimidate to a certain degree, as if associating with a disabled cancer survivor somehow transmits the disease. Although I am sure this is not a universal truth, it has been my experience that cancer survivors make grateful, appreciative people, if not too embittered by the effects wrought on them by their condition. It is worth spending the time to ascertain how that person, if they're in your life, would like to be treated and base your actions on how you yourself would seek to be treated. I would suggest understanding and patience are good places to start, and all the more so since current statistics reflect that one in four of us will be touched by cancer of some form or another.

Chapter Nine

A Matter of Microbes

Music: *Mozart, Sonata in E-Flat, K. 282,*
played by Sviatoslav Richter

After about a decade of dressing my leaking leg, I must have
tried every conceivable type of gauze, bandage and attachment
method. Constantly aware that my skin was in bad shape, I
consulted regularly with my pharmacist to try new approaches.
On one occasion, it was suggested I attach a colostomy bag
to the sinus with the most discharge and leave it in situ until
it was full of the grim green gunk. This was slightly better that
having leakage through my trousers. However, on removing
the colostomy bag, the adhesive took a considerable amount of
skin with it, so this idea was abandoned. In the end, the most
enduringly useful configuration was a combination of the usual
gauze pads held in place by elasticated stocking material. If the
family was on holiday, we'd always be accompanied by a suitcase
exclusively for dressings and medications, as if we had an extra
family member; in this case, a colony of microbes – a permanent,
unbidden guest until the next surgery.

At follow-up sessions with the Stanmore team, the question
was always about when I'd had enough of the situation and
wanted to come in for another revision.

By this time, I was under the care of the Aston team. Mr Will Aston, a consultant orthopaedic surgeon, was a new face to me. I was immediately impressed by his calm demeanour and softly-spoken manner, which instilled me with the necessary confidence to proceed. I agreed that enough was indeed enough and so I was officially listed for surgery. I had become used to the idea that this next surgical phase would be far from straightforward due to the infection. As if on cue, from the time of the decision to proceed, the output from the leaks increased considerably. We had to hope that the infection would not go systemic via the bloodstream and set up other sites throughout my body. Apparently, as I later discovered, I had been under constant threat from septicaemia. Perhaps antibiotics had staved off the activities of the infection but they would never kill it. Surgery was essential.

✶✶✶✶✶

The plan was to go in through the existing scar site, remove the prosthesis and clean out whatever was found to be dwelling in my tissues, cutting away as little of the remaining bone as possible. We hoped that there would be enough left to make a further revision possible. If not then amputation would be the only course. Upon removal of the metalwork, a temporary spacer would be loosely cemented in. Impregnated with antibiotics, the action would be twofold; to kill off any remaining infection and to maintain the shape and functionality of my leg itself. After enough of an interval and subject to the blood-borne infection markers decreasing to an acceptable level, there would be another operation, similar to this last one. It would involve removing the spacer and inserting a definitive prosthesis, permanently cemented in this time. A course of intense, targeted, intravenous antibiotics would follow for as long as it took to achieve the desired blood count. Memories of lying in bed like Da Vinci's 'Vitruvian Man' were soon supplanted by the news that these drugs would be administered at home every day through a line going directly into my heart. Thankfully, the injections would be done by a visiting district nurse. I'd heard of this technique for administering drugs via a Hickman line and always dreaded having one. My overwhelming thought was whether I'd be able to feel weird sensations in my chest as cold drugs were pumped in, and whether I'd be able to feel the tube inside my heart. Speculation like this is not useful. As on many occasions before, I decided to take it as it would come, and be grateful that this new treatment was around and could give me a chance at recovery.

It was a while since I'd been in Stanmore for surgery. Little had changed with the infrastructure – the place still looked rather like the collection of derelict dormitories it always had. Strangely comforting, although a shaming indictment of the lack of funding to this incredible place. My wife and I stayed in the Spartan accommodation offered for families the night before the operation. I was scheduled to be available from 7a.m. the following morning and felt that some sleep before surgery would be good. I slept like a baby; my wife understandably could not and kept an uneasy vigil.

I duly checked in at the ward, nil by mouth since the evening before, gagging for tea and wondering how long it would be before I could enjoy that lovely liquid coursing down my throat. When you can't have something, your desire for it increases exponentially. I made myself comfortable in my surgical gown, open to the elements at the back, and tried to doze off. Although it was now 28 years after my first knee surgery, and a lot had happened (albeit unexpectedly) in the intervening years, here I was again; stuck on a hospital bed, waiting. In my current state, that is to say divested of my habitual clothing, wedding ring, signet ring, I looked down at my beleaguered leg and thought about the story that my body could tell; scars, wasted muscles, leaking holes, dodgy back and a return to baldness, not this time by chemotherapy drugs but by the attrition of age and genetics. It's a time like this that you inevitably reflect on what your life actually means in the grand scheme of it all. I ran various memories through my mind, mostly of being with my wife and children on holiday and days out, laughing, eating together, Christmases, birthdays. I thought about the long document I'd written and deposited with my brother-in-law, Jonathan, and also with our family solicitor.

I called it my 'Disaster Letter'; a kind of take care of business letter if I didn't get off the operating table, if all that was left of me was memories in other people's minds and a big chunk of old metalwork. I didn't feel morbid about it. After all, life had been absolutely fantastic, cancer notwithstanding, up to that very moment. I had nothing to regret. I had everything to live for and wanted to. Very badly. Every other thought receded and I remembered the strange calm, limbo-like place I was able to get to from before. Not long afterwards, I was called for and the theatre porters arrived, jocular but professional. The theatre nurse assigned to me came and checked me over for metalwork, dentures and piercings. The only thing that concerned me was that the big, thick black arrow on my left leg was clearly visible. The encouraging calls from fellow patients started as I was wheeled out on the bed. Nods, winks, the odd call of 'All the best, mate' were very welcome.

In the ante-room, I met the anaesthetist again, and we continued a bizarre conversation about the band Hawkwind, which we'd started earlier on the ward.

A plastic blanket was placed over me and started to inflate with warm air. A new pre-surgical preparation technique, I assumed. Hopefully this would make my veins conspicuous enough so that I wouldn't need another needle in the neck. To the sound in my mind of the intro to *Masters of the Universe* and curiously remembering that it was once used as the introduction to a school assembly back at St Clement Danes of all places, I tried to follow the instruction to count down from 10, and failed.

*****

The space was immense, suffused in a golden glow. Tremulous strings, low horns intoning a two-note rhythm like a slow and purposeful knock. After a pause, the rhythm is back this time, moving up from D to F and back. Minor thirds, fifths, D minor, and as the strings swell, the key note D splits into C# and D#... I become aware that I am conducting the opening of Bruckner's *Ninth Symphony* and aware that the horns are actually me, bellowing. The light turns strongly white, I feel like my arms are getting ready to give an appropriately colossal downbeat on a massive B major chord...

'Fre-ed,' the sing-song call of the nurse penetrated the Brucknerian nimbus. The strong light was issuing from above my bed in the recovery room.

'Ahhhhhh! My thumb!' I felt as if my left thumb was being squeezed hard and ever harder in a vice.

'What's he saying?' the nurse asked my wife, who I realised was now at the bedside.

'It's the clip on his thumb, can we take it off? He broke his thumb. It's from a car crash and is on the list to be repaired.'

We later had a good laugh about me waking up from major leg surgery, the removal and replacement of a grossly-infected metal component, to complain about a broken thumb clamped in an oxygenation reader!

I asked my wife how long I'd been out and knowing me very well, she replied that she'd already asked if I could have a cup of tea. I was not allowed this mercy until I'd stopped feeling nauseous and when it eventually arrived, I took small sips through a straw, as administered by my wife. I was told I could control my pain by squeezing on a button I was holding in my right hand. This would pump a small but significant dose of morphine straight into my system – like being immersed in a warm bath. Once I began to be able to put some thoughts together in some kind of order, I realised that I couldn't feel much going on in the leg department. I dreaded to look but when I finally managed it, I could see toes sticking out of the end of the sheet covering me. See but not yet feel. Fortified by more sips of that heavenly liquid, I resolved not to use the morphine button until I felt something from the leg, and is wasn't long before I did. A slight tingle grew into a sensation of heavy immobility, soon followed by searing pain. This was good news to me. I tried to flex the muscles. When I couldn't tolerate how much it was hurting, I hit the 'warm bath' button and drifted back into Bruckner-land.

Waking up back on the ward, my wife was with me and she told me I was in one piece. I looked at my left leg, heavily bandaged underneath a substantial black brace, and with the familiar sight of two drains leading away to blood-filled bottles secured to the side of the bedframe. A gloriously golden brown piece of toast appeared, with more tea.

Soon afterwards, we saw the surgical team, who were pleased with the procedure. I am glad they did not go into too many specifics right there and then – I was able later to read the specific record of the operation in magnificent detail. Certain phrases would have been more at home in a script for the *Saw* movie franchise. The less said, the better. I received instructions not to move the leg. The spacer was only loosely cemented in as it would be coming back out again relatively soon. I was to avoid bending at the knee (hence the brace) and avoid weight-bearing. Even at this stage, there were still significant risks and I wasn't clear of the woods yet. In addition to the need for extreme care, when I could finally move around, I had the new daily rigour of intravenous antibiotics once again. For the moment, these were administered in the conventional way. Later, I would be fitted with the line into my heart. The specific drugs had been tailored by a new team of microbiologists working at Stanmore, led by Dr Simon Warren, to provide antibiotic cover. This would be the all-important statistical indicator. If the C-reactive protein number started descending from its current level at around 26 then that part of the outcome would be successful. Quite a few factors had to go well in order for this to have worked. I became mentally exhausted by just thinking about this. Pervading all of this was my greater concern for my wife and children. I had to be as strong as possible for them. I remain optimistically jocular by nature and fully espouse the doctrine first articulated by Timon in *The Lion King* – *Hakuna Matata* or, for the uninitiated, *No Worries*. Of course, it went without saying that my children in particular knew why their dad was in hospital, having lived with my orthopaedic problems most of their own lives. Indeed, my youngest had never known me as an able-bodied person. She must have believed that my crutches were permanently attached as I hadn't been able to get around without them for years. I decided that the main priorities were to follow the guidance of the surgeons, physios and nurses, keep still as directed, and eat as well as I could. In addition to the excellent provisions at RNOH, my wife had brought in, at my request, my stash of super-food supplements; aloe vera juice, a jar of malt extract (not to be confused with the single, liquid, Scottish variety of malt), various nuts, seeds, cranberries, dried apricots, figs and chocolate, all of which found their way into the morning porridge in ritualistic fashion. The cranberries were to prevent any kind of problems with 'male plumbing', figs and apricots to fulfil their alimentary mission in relation to ease of digestive transit. I had to wait and see if my much-damaged body still had sufficient powers of recuperation. The surgeons had a great phrase for this: 'Mr Scott, your muscles have suffered great insult,' this truth delivered with sensitive diplomacy.

It was very important to me to make sure I was eating as much as possible in order to make sure my 'insulted' body was getting fuel. In this regard, I was extremely grateful for the three hot meals, every day, served with great cheerfulness by our Filipina catering manager on the ward. This, and my supply of nuts and fruit, helped me to believe I was nourishing the parts that most required it. This, and regular encounters with chemically-enhanced *Mozart Adagios* on CD kept me going.

My wife had once again to make regularly the long journey from South London up to Stanmore. A major imposition, I felt, but it's hard to express how wonderful it always was to see her come, always smiling, down the long corridor of the ward. When I knew a few days later that she was bringing my youngest in, I vowed to myself that I would be standing when they arrived. I desperately did not want my daughter to see me horizontal. No matter what it took, I would be upright. The physiotherapy team at Stanmore worked wonders and had me upright about two days after the operation. Discomfort aside, and although wondering if my bones would take it, standing with crutches was not that difficult. I was rather shaky and dizzy, not allowed to put any weight through the left leg, but more or less upright. We practiced getting off the bed, bearing in mind I was still hooked up to drains and drips, and managed to negotiate a journey to the day room, all of 10 steps. So, when I knew my wife and daughter had arrived, I made it up and stood at the end of my bed, waiting.

My wife and daughters look almost identical, albeit at different ages, and have identical smiles. This sight, even from the distance of 30 or so metres, made me want to laugh, cry, shout out with joy and weep like a baby. I held on for the sake of my ward-mates and kept a measure of control. That hug was the sweetest gift and like a reward for having been chopped around again. When my eldest arrived back from university for a visit, I was equally overjoyed to see her. The last time I'd had a protracted stay here, she'd been seven years old. And now here she was, a grown woman, a phenomenal singer, beautiful and confident. We sat and talked, holding hands for hours. My son came at the weekend and spent a day with me, watching DVDs and joking around in his inimitable, dry way. Mature and brave way beyond his years, he had been four years old last time I'd been in RNOH. Here he was now, a tall, handsome, young man of great musical accomplishments with a keen mind and tested through severe trials of his own. The love of my family was the greatest single factor in my recovery and determination to get out and back home. However, that could not have happened without the unprecedented expertise of the incomprehensibly patient and kind nursing staff on the ward.

These professionals could never be remunerated close to their true worth to people like me. Something else drives them. Lugman, Edna, Lisia, Kalpana and many others exemplify all that's good about humanity. Prepared to meet you at the point of your greatest vulnerability, they bring you up again. Every observations round was an event to me. I wanted to follow those stats very closely, asking about temperature and blood pressure obsessively. Any rise in temperature could indicate infection. There were frequent blood tests measuring the CRP. This was lowering all too slowly. Any spike upwards would be bad news. CRP can indicate infection and also shows due to surgical trauma – a double-whammy. I had to focus on the second part of that and believe that the infection had been significantly challenged by the surgery. The thrice-daily antibiotic IVs must have been doing something too. This regime had been crafted by the new microbiology team and was specific to the bugs that had made my leg their home until now. I discussed my special recipe of supplements with the various staff members and interestingly to me, the Pharmacist was particularly supportive of my use of aloe vera, malt extract, nuts, seeds and cranberry juice, which I consumed in great quantities, determined to stave off any and every type of infection known to man. After about 10 days of this routine, the surgeons were happy for me to go home. Infection markers were on the way down and the physios had made sure I had enough confidence and a clear understanding of the parameters of movement allowed. One thing remained – to have a Hickman line inserted into my heart.

The thought is bad enough and it's impossible not to speculate about feeling things crawling around inside your chest cavity. My imagination was lively on this subject to say the least. I realised that I'd become somewhat inured to the thought and consequences of major surgery. It was the ancillary procedures that made me feel most uncomfortable. The insertion was not done at the bedside as I'd imagined, but in a sort of operating room by a team of three. I remember light-hearted banter with the technician and nurse before meeting the consultant, who explained that he'd pass some local anaesthetic in and thread the catheter into my heart via my left arm. By now, I'd had countless injections and my fears about the viability of my damaged veins were allayed by the team and within minutes, the tube was in, perfectly painlessly. It was slightly surreal to think that the end of the tube attached to my left arm created an open aperture right into what is arguably the most important organ in the human body. I learned that I would be visited daily at home by district nurses, who would monitor my wound, do blood tests, and inject the all-important antibiotics.

After discharge and the drive home through Central London traffic, I settled in and took stock of the situation. I felt fragile and tentative. The road ahead looked impossibly long. I could barely stand, every movement accompanied by breath-taking pain, a weak and depleted body enveloped in a cloud of exhaustion. At least, I reflected, things could only improve from this baseline. With that cheery thought, I drifted off to sleep, looking at the welcome home cards from my children. It's impossible to catalogue the vast number of scenarios that play out in your mind during recovery. I had been here a few times now so to a certain extent, I knew what to expect and how to deal with it; rest, eat a lot, take the medicine, and keep the mind active and stimulated, looking forwards.

*****

The next day saw the beginning of the daily visits of the district nurses to monitor my wounds and inject me with the antibiotics. I was so encouraged by the sensitivity and expertise of these professionals as they went about their undeniably unpleasant business. My scar looked horrendous; a long reddy-pink ridge, traversed by metal clips like large staples holding it all together.

Memories of the last time when it all split open came to mind. I could foresee much pain when these clips had to be removed. In the quietness of home, I was more tuned in to how my body was feeling, all the discomforts and signals of distress from various places. The moment arrived for the injection into the heart. I must admit that I'd been imagining this and was prepared for some strange sensations. In the event, I suppose due to a lack of the right kind of nerve cells in those blood vessels, there was no icy cold flood into my chest after all. When it was finished, the nurse left, saying I was doing well so far. We'd wait to see if the infection indicators were heading downwards before getting too excited. After all, if they weren't, I'd be back up to Stanmore soon. Much as I appreciated the place, I wanted to put some space between me and the establishment, at least for a while.

About an hour or so after the injection, I began to feel truly dreadful, reminiscent of the old chemo treatments. Although I felt like it, there was no throwing up, just a deep and abiding nausea, dizziness and disorientation. This was to last several hours. I figured that if the drugs could make me feel this terrible, they must be annihilating the bacteria in a big way. So this was to be the new pattern of my days; a few good hours in the late afternoon and evening, trying to find a reasonably comfortable position for sleeping, and the knowledge that the next day I'd spend a good deal of it feeling atrocious. I'd become slightly obsessive about the markers, knowing that a successful outcome rather hinged on their consistent lowering. Thankfully, this was to be the case and for this, I am indebted to the fantastic work of the Stanmore microbiologists. I now had the all-clear to be listed for the definitive knee replacement, which would remove the spacer and refit me with a fully-cemented, permanent prosthesis. How in the world this could possibly work, again, was beyond my ability to comprehend. Four knee replacements on the same side. Maybe a record of some kind? That aside, I was wondering how much more serious aggravation my bones and muscles could endure at the age of 52.

Chapter Ten

Home Straight

Music: *The Donor – Judee Sill*

Within a few months, I was back in, re-admitted for what I was hoping would be the final operation in this series. Back on the same ward, seeing familiar faces among the nursing staff, with one exception. During my previous stay, one of the most caring of the nurses had, unbeknownst to many of her colleagues, received a diagnosis of breast cancer herself. Continuing to work until she was unable to carry on, she had recently died. She had decided to help as many as possible, despite her own affliction. This was shocking and sad but a reason for me to commemorate her here and request that nursing staff are recognised not only for what they are seen to do but what they personally sacrifice in order to care for us. It is certainly not a profession that one enters for remunerative gain. So many more unworthy individuals are over-compensated for far less positive impact on humanity. It always seems to me quite shaming that those tasked with administering the nation's healthcare seem so unable or unwilling to ensure that this crucial role is at least a financially viable career option. How much longer can we rely purely on the good will and altruistic impulse of those that would care for us despite this? Surely the time has come for talking and agonising to cease and for simple decisions to be made boldly to rectify this travesty while time remains. Perhaps a spell in hospital shadowing a healthcare professional would serve to illustrate the point. I seriously wonder if any of our political class would be courageous or imaginative enough to do this without the inevitable photo-opportunity as motivation. It is an election year, at the time of writing, so who knows?

The day for surgery had arrived. Nil by mouth, checklist done, wedding ring taped up, surgical gown on, big arrow on left leg – I was ready.

'Ten, nine, eight, sev...'

*****

I was back again in the huge and expansive place of the golden glow.

This time, I was surrounded by the music of Bach – the magnificent *B minor Mass*. The opening Kyrie's fugue, a very chromatic, semi-tone rich theme, which the great Johann Sebastian was able to weave and build like a cosmos. I became part of this. I heard a voice and felt it emanating from my chest, the entry of the basses, then...

'Fr-ed. How do you feel?'

I was back in recovery, not actually in paradise after all. A wave of warmth and I was out again, back to the place of the golden glow. Low strings moving upwards in steps in a triplet rhythm. Again a choir, male voices. The final movement of the Busoni *Piano Concerto*. I am conducting, singing along with the choir in the final hymn section of the movement.

'Why's he waving his arms around?'

'He always does this after surgery.' It's the voice of my wife, explaining to the recovery nurse my usual post-op behaviour.

The impact on those waiting for someone who's in surgery cannot be underestimated. They had told her that I would be gone for around four to five hours. Previously, she had watched the clock to the minute and had become progressively and understandably more anxious every minute past the allotted time. After this particular operation, my wife knew that the timing was approximate. Waiting on the ward until she was called by recovery, she came along. As she was just about to enter the room, the demeanour of the nurse changed as she said, 'Sorry. Something's wrong. You need to wait outside. You can't be in this area now!' Immediately, she assumed that I was crashing. She was allowed in after the incident had resolved. A fellow recovery patient had been vomiting after waking up. After she had been allowed in, it was apparently reassuring for her to hear me loudly singing Busoni's great hymn.

*****

Within two days, I was sitting on the bed and for the first time in many years, I was able to bend my left leg to 90 degrees, and there it was, hanging over the side of the bed. The mandatory blood drains still attached, I was up and walking around on my Zimmer frame, even allowed to start putting a little weight through the left leg too. A day or so later, and with the consent of the surgical team, I was moved to Jubilee Ward; a new rehabilitation programme for post-operative patients in a low-maintenance environment. The regime was somewhat more relaxed. One of the great benefits was a communal eating room where we could eat together and talk. The atmosphere was rather like a pub but without the alcohol. All of the chaps were recently operated on and soon to be discharged.

Visiting hours were very flexible and daily visits were divided up between my two older children, my wife and youngest, and also my best friend from our Royal Academy days, Louis Demetrius Alvanis. Although we are about as different as it is possible to be in many ways, Louis and I have remained close friends since we first met at RAM back in 1979. His extraordinary brilliance as a pianist is rightly recognised around the world. As fathers of three children, we have much in common.

My eldest daughter came over one evening for a very welcome visit. We sat in this large communal television room watching some or other non-descript reality TV nonsense and enjoying a takeaway together. She was going to stay over in the family accommodation so we talked until late. My first child, and now an adult. I remembered keenly the moment when her mother announced that she thought she might be pregnant way back in 1993. It had been a very difficult time with the recent death of my father from cancer. He was much reduced by his disease and, unable to eat, had diminished in stature alarmingly. Unable to stand, he took great pleasure in demonstrating how he could turn his bedside television on and off with his walking stick. The last time I saw him, I estimated he must have weighed no more than 50 kg, if that. This contradicted all my memories of him and his impressive physical strength, which had persisted until the final days of his cancer. About nine months after his death, my daughter was born. As I sat with her that night up at Stanmore, I reflected how proud of her my father would be. He had spent his working life at Covent Garden, very close to the Royal Opera House. It is an almost unbearable thought that he was never able in this life to hear his granddaughter sing the operatic arias he loved, nor indeed the music his grandson had composed, which had been regularly used at the Opera House and broadcast on BBC radio.

My mother followed him six years later. Driving with her one day, I asked if she was lonely.

'No one's asked me that. And I really am.' It was heart-breaking to feel her loss after over 50 years together with my father. We drove and talked about him. Although it was somewhat consoling for both of us, I knew that this had been a catastrophic loss for her. I had come in one evening from work when my wife, looking ashen, asked me to sit down. She told me my mother had died on the way to hospital after a heart attack. It was some consolation that she'd had a chance to see both of my older children, but a bitter disappointment that she, as a relative of the great Marie Lloyd, quite possibly the most famous female Music Hall singer, the Madonna of her time, had never heard her granddaughter sing.

As I looked at my lovely daughter, I was overwhelmingly thankful. Here was an affirmation of life in the midst of all this death. For me, it was a challenge to resolve to get over the latest operation as quickly as I could and get back to the business of living.

Three days later, I was able to go home.

*****

A few follow-up visits from the district nurse, one of which was to remove the metal staples securing my scar (45 individual episodes of sharp pain) came and went quickly. I started having regular physiotherapy sessions at RNOH Bolsover Street and gained more confidence in movement during these visits, under the guidance of Ollie Cowper, who has essentially taught me how to walk again. For the first time in many years, I am not applying dressings to the two leaking holes on my leg. The skills of Mr

Aston and his team put an end to those. I now have two circular patches that resemble gunshot wounds, adding to the dramatic scar itself, which had been opened for all the previous operations.

Since the infection has been dealt with, I have received interesting reactions from people who knew me during that period, usually centring around the fact that I look very well and healthy these days instead of terribly sick, drawn and other similarly descriptive epithets. It's great to hear in retrospect how people really perceive you when you're ill. All the medical professionals I see these days look ridiculously young to me. Perhaps it's the cliché inherent in the typical middle-aged observation that your own physical youth has gone. I just cannot get beyond believing that I'm still about 23 years old though. Of course, the intervening years have taken a massive toll if I stop to think about it; seven major operations, seven general anaesthetics, hours and hours of controlled unconsciousness at the edge of death, scores of accumulated X-rays, gamma rays, CAT scans, MRI scans, ultrasounds, blood tests, antibiotics, painkillers, not to mention the horrendous chemotherapy drugs themselves, and all the hours of physiotherapy, the painful process of learning to walk again a few extra times. Even today, there is a background of constant pain as a legacy. Sometimes I'm convinced my memory isn't all it should be. I can memorise music as I always could, but it's the fact that I often find myself, to the amusement of my family, asking them the same things over and over again. I count myself fortunate to have the kind of temperament that likes a fight, although I cannot honestly say I started out that way. If it doesn't kill you... as they say.

*****

We planned a family holiday to Sardinia and for once, we didn't have to lug around a suitcase full of dressings for my leaking leg. In the blazing heat of that fabulous place, I had a little time to reflect back on the years of relentless fighting, pushing, striving. Floating in the transparent sea, not having to worry about the previous routine of applying layers of waterproof dressings, I looked up to the clear blue sky, the blazing sun recharging my spirit. No wonder it was worshipped as a deity. A water-wrestling match with my son brings me back to reality.

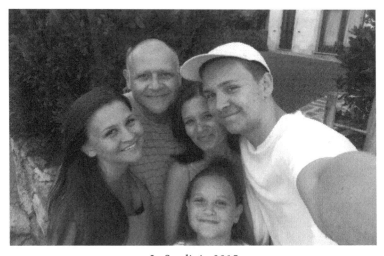

In Sardinia 2015

'I'm stronger than you, old man!' Yes he is. I'm grateful for that, to be able to hear him say it, to see him bronzed by the sun. Looking back to the beach, I see the other pillars of my world, my wife and daughters. I walk out of the sea to embrace them. Their love warms me more than the sun.

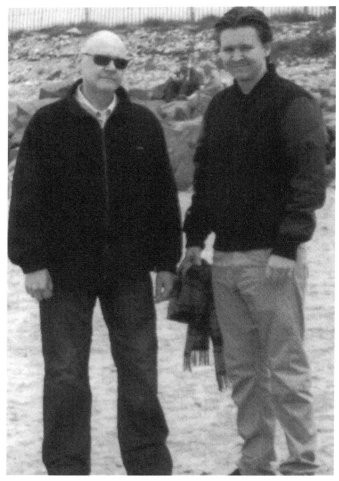

Father and son, North Norfolk coast, 2015

This is the story so far. There is no proper final chapter yet. No conclusion. In this uncharted territory, life goes on.

I've been alive for 54 years now, 30 of those, the majority, as someone living with cancer. Not a disease inflicted from outside but an organic part of me, like blue eyes, male pattern baldness, destined to show itself sooner or later due to a peculiarity of my genes.

Maybe one day, I'll feel my age.

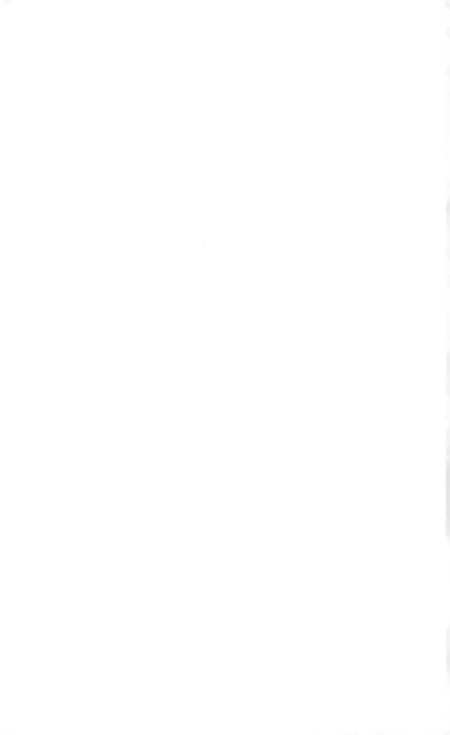

Epilogue

Music: *Here I Am – Bryan Adams*

It was an autumnal morning, soggy with rainfall. The characteristic aroma of damp leaves, the sound of ducks, geese and parakeets in the air around us. For the first time, I had ventured out of the car to take a few steps without my walking stick. Since it was early, my leg was not yet too tired or painful to hold me up on its own. I was in our favourite local park with my youngest. She has the irrepressible energy of her age and the luminous curiosity of wonder about nature. She runs on ahead, of course with the understanding that she cannot go beyond my line of sight, and runs back to report on the situation of the Mandarin ducks and Canada geese. We have brought a bag of peanuts in their shells and are looking out for squirrels. It is not long before they appear, hesitant, bouncing around, snuffling among fallen leaves.

'These guys do NOT have great eyesight!' I say, as we throw down nuts for them. They seem not to bother looking where the nuts land but rather find them by sense of smell. We listen in rapt awe to the tiny crunching sounds as the squirrels de-shell the peanuts and run up trees to savour the contents before returning for another. My daughter ventures on, stopping to ask owners if she might stroke their dogs as they walk them. Everyone is friendly, indulgent. There's a kind of fellowship among the park crowd at this time of day.

I ask her questions about the different types of birds and she can tell me all about them, their diet, habitat, migratory predilections, everything.

I cannot be happier, more fulfilled, loving life – the pain and challenges eclipsed by this experience. My little girl is at the riverbank, she turns and walks a little slower than usual back towards me, an idyllic smile on her face. She walks right up to me and nuzzles her head against my amply-upholstered middle, putting her arms around me. Looking up, she says, 'I love you, Daddy. I just wanted to tell you.' A squeeze, and off she runs again, chasing a pigeon.

*****

Musical Appendix

Prologue

Can You Feel the Groove Tonight – Con Funk Shun

I first heard this on the Greg Edwards funk and soul show on Capital Radio. Greg described it as the 'the real funk, as it is, as it was, as it always should be'.

At this particular point in life, I was putting in as many hours as I could physically handle, learning and practicing new piano repertoire by day and spending long hours at night writing music. In the 1980s, there was a burgeoning funk and jazz-funk scene in the UK. I was introduced by a school friend to Joe Zawinul's Weather Report, featuring the uniquely virtuosic bass-playing of Jaco Pastorius. Remembering regular trips to the Half-Moon pub in Putney to hear Morrissey-Mullen still fills me with nostalgia for a great era in music. *Can You Feel the Groove* encapsulates it all.

Chapter One – Water on the Knee

Torna a Sorriento – Luciano Pavarotti

From a fine album of Neapolitan songs, sung with grandeur and emotion. It takes about two notes to know you're hearing this great tenor. The powerfully sentimental music always filled me with overwhelming optimism at a time when I didn't yet have any particular cares in the world.

Chapter Two – An Ending and a Beginning

Beethoven; *Piano Sonata in C Minor Op. 111* – Wilhelm Kempff

About as great as it gets, Kempff, Master-Beethovenian in the ultimate realisation of this music. Tremendous anticipation and later turbulence resolve into complete peace.

I was fortunate enough to hear this superb artist at the Royal Festival Hall in the 1980s. My piano teacher, Mrs Creighton, took me to hear all the great pianists of that time; Sviatoslav Richter, Emil Gilels, Vladimir Horowitz, Claudio Arrau, Arturo Benedetti Michelangeli and Shura Cherkassky, to name a few. These concerts are etched in my mind to this day, as is the visionary generosity of my teacher.

She died last year, aged 102, and it had been my privilege to play for her whenever I visited. I had regularly sent her videos and recordings from wherever I was performing. I cannot fully express what she did for me. Her photograph is near my teaching piano and I am thankful every day.

Chapter Three – Death Row

Give Blood – Pete Townshend

It just seemed to fit at the time – powerful, pounding and doom-laden, yielding to major mode optimism.

I had listened to the music of The Who since primary school days. Having older siblings meant that I had always been listening to their music, which ranged from the blues of Sonny Boy Williamson and Louisiana Red, cutting-edge jazz of Ornette Coleman via Frank Zappa and the Mothers of Invention, to Jimi Hendrix, Cream, James Taylor and Joni Mitchell. Two of my older siblings worked at Sound City, where a lot of these musicians bought their instruments and played seminal gigs nearby at the

Marquee in Soho. My own musical interests extended to Emerson, Lake and Palmer, Yes and Pink Floyd. My influential brother-in-law introduced me to The Who and later, Pete Townshend's solo albums. *Give Blood* from his *White City* album just seemed to be an anthem for me at the time.

Chapter Four – 'We Can Re-build Him'

Training Montage from Rocky IV – Vince di Cola

Di Cola's innovative use of the Fairlight synthesiser was revolutionary. You cannot hear this irresistible track and not feel it's the perfect accompaniment to physical struggle.

Orthopaedic surgery always requires a certain amount of re-training and physiotherapy to regain useful function. Little did I know, during my carefree days at the gym, how hard I would need to work just to get up and stand up after each subsequent operation. This particular music will make anyone feel they can do anything!

Chapter Five – Ramble On

The Song Remains the Same – Led Zeppelin

This is rather like a hymn to the omnipresence and omniscience of music and how it pervades life.

I have always listened to Led Zeppelin, and this particular song encapsulates the significance of my re-engagement with the world of music when I was feeling that it had gone from my life for good.

As Robert Plant sings, '*Any little song that you know... Everything that's small has to grow*'.

Chapter Six – Love of My Life

Through The Fire – Chaka Khan
What would you risk for The One?

I played this song to my future wife when I was giving her a lift in my car one evening. I put the tape on and ducked out to buy a bottle of water in a corner shop near Munster Road in Fulham, leaving just enough time for Chaka to communicate what I was thinking and hoping desperately she would work her magic!

Chapter Seven – 'We Can Revise Him'

Symphony no 4 'Det Uudslukkelige' – Carl Nielsen
Defiant and life-affirming, written in 1916, when the world was seemingly falling apart.

I had this symphony almost on a loop at the time. Nielsen's sublime music gave me resolve during a particularly hard time in Stanmore. It expresses, as he said, 'the elemental will to live'.

Chapter Eight – 2001 – Beyond The Millennium

Symphonia from *Doktor* Faust – Ferruccio Busoni
Busoni, a futuristic composer, who wrote for a 'future that has yet to arrive', as pianist Arthur Loesser said.

My first encounter with arguably the most significant composer to span the late-Romantic and Modern eras came at my piano teacher's house. From where I used to sit at her Bechstein grand piano, I could see her immense record collection to my left, in cabinets behind where she would sit for our lessons. The spine of one particular boxed set of records bore the names 'Busoni' and '*Doktor Faust*' in old German script. Captivated by the look of it, I asked her what this was. This led me to borrow the opera.

From the very first two-note chord of the *Symphonia*, I was then, and have remained, captivated by Busoni's unique sound world. This music is like an appeal to the future; his personal philosophy was 'always look ahead'.

Chapter Nine – *A Matter of Microbes*

Mozart; *Piano Sonata in E-Flat, K.282* – Sviatoslav Richter

Mozart's exquisite adagio first movement, played by the Colossus of the piano.

Richter was Mrs Creighton's favourite pianist, and she took me to hear him several times at the Royal Festival Hall. Each experience was and remains unforgettable. No one living or dead could make a mere construction of metal and wood live and breathe as he did. The sheer physical force of Richter's musical personality could be felt like a breaking wave as he walked briskly to the piano. The atmosphere created by thousands of audience members in totally breathless silence before the opening 5th of Schubert's *Sonata in A Minor, Op. 143* was a spectacle of cosmic proportion.

Chapter Ten – *Home Straight*

The Donor – Judee Sill

'Kyrie Eleison' – one of the truest representations of spiritual ecstasy in music or any other art form for that matter.

It's true that 'neglected' artists have sometimes earned their neglect by being mediocre. Nothing is further from the truth for Judee Sill. I was watching a re-run of Bob Harris's *Old Grey Whistle Test* a few years ago when he introduced a studio performance given by Judee in London. The song, *The Kiss* was unlike anything I had heard. Her short and tragic life took her off the scene that became the province of the great female singer/ songwriters. She has the right to be counted alongside the other great genius composers who were taken too soon. Along with Mozart and Schubert, Judee Sill's creativity burned brightly for less than 40 years in life, but her music still illuminates the world she left behind. Listening to this wonderful song after surgery, I was immersed in feelings of relief and thankfulness, accompanied by tears.

Epilogue

Here I Am – Bryan Adams

My youngest daughter sings and embodies this song about the wildness and freedom of the Spirit.

A keen rider, she tells me that when on horseback, she feels completely free and alive. The closest I come to that is when I'm playing or composing music. That autumnal morning was my new day, my new start.